NUTRITION AND THE ATHLETE

NUTRITION AND THE ATHLETE

Joseph J. Morella
and
Richard J. Turchetti

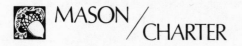 MASON/CHARTER

NEW YORK 1976

Library of Congress Cataloging in Publication Data

Morella, Joseph J   1939–
  Nutrition and the athlete.

  Includes index.
  1. Athletes—Nutrition.   I. Turchetti,
Richard J., 1940–   joint author. II. Title.
TX361.A8M67   641.1′02′4796   76–1940
ISBN 0–88405–132–3
ISBN 0–88405–120–X pbk.

CONTENTS

WITH FONDEST APPRECIATION AND LOVE TO
MARILYN FEELY, ELAINE TURCHETTI, DICK HAMM,
TONY GAROFANO, AND JERRY KATZ.

1 INTRODUCTION

Throughout man's history there has been an emphasis on the development of physical culture. Physical fitness is not only an expression of physical exercise for recreational purposes. There has always been a direct relationship between people's fitness and their ability to withstand the strain and stresses of their environment. The aphorism "survival of the fittest" proves to be the natural law for evolutionary growth. It is necessary, therefore, to trace through the past to extract information on contemporary attitudes concerning man and athletics.

Empirical facts have illustrated that man in his most primitive states prepared himself physically for the arduous hunt for food and the battle with hostile neighbors. Often these preparations were subsequently turned into rituals in the form of dances, ceremonies, and the like.

Superstition and magic gave birth to the ideas that alterations in diet enhanced physical output. Some primitive people thought that swallowing powdered lions' teeth imparted the strength of the animal. Others believed that devouring animal hearts or similar organs conferred the particular virtue that animal represented. In some primitive societies these customs persist.

Ancient Greece spawned the concept that "muscle meat" endowed its taker with "muscle" strength. Prior to this belief, formulated by Dromeus of Stymphalus (450 B.C.), an athlete's diet was traditionally vegetarian, containing only the smallest amount of meat. Dromeus believed that since "muscle" was so extensively used in athletic pursuits, athletes should logi-

cally replenish "muscle" substance by eating "more muscle,"
or greater amounts of meat, thereby becoming better athletes. As it happened, his athletes were already genetically
superior. When they began eating heavy meat diets and were
successful, the people incorrectly assumed heavy meat eating
(high protein intake) had a direct relationship to strength and
endurance. Even today there are athletes and coaches who
swear by a meat-dominated, heavy protein diet for maximum
strength and efficiency.

Physical culture played an important part in the development of the Greek city-states. This is indicated most strongly
in the Minoan and Hellenic cultures, where the upper classes
were the group from which warriors were drawn. Until almost the present day physical culture has been largely
confined to the higher social classes.

In the later Hellenic period physical education spread
from the city-state elite to the entire population as a treatment for disease and disability. The medical application of
athletics was promoted during the Roman Empire by Galen,
who served as both team physician to the gladiators and athletes and as personal physician to Marcus Aurelius.

Throughout the centuries athletes have been held by society to be the epitomes of health and vigor. The athlete—"the
fittest"—has survived and endured better than the average
man. The struggle for existence today is no less arduous than
it was 5,000 years ago—however, instead of famines, hostile
neighbors, wild animals, and the elements modern man must
fight pollution, emotional stress, and technological shock. The
survival of the fittest theory is as valid today as it ever was.
Well-fed, athletic people are obviously the "fittest."

Considering the fact that both athletics and nutrition are
two subjects that have interested people for centuries, it is
amazing how little information has been compiled concerning
the effects of nutrition on physical fitness and performance.
It was not until the late eighteenth century, when there was
a rapid growth of interest in sports in England, that observers
became concerned with the athletic diet.

It was customary early in the nineteenth century for the athlete to begin his training with a series of strong purges to clear away "the noxious matter he may have had in his stomach and intestines." Following this "purification," mild beer, bread, and underdone, unseasoned red meat were prescribed. An article in *Lancet*, the British medical journal, states that

> The Oxford crew in the 1860's trained on a diet of underdone beef or mutton, bread, tea and beer, with a little jelly or watercress as a treat at the evening meal. Instructions were given that no vegetables were to be eaten. Cambridge, on the other hand, suffered no restrictions regarding potatoes, greens, or even fruit. From 1861 to 1869 there was an unbroken succession of Oxford victories.

Although there has been some interest in the athlete's diet and training, it has been limited to those directly concerned with athletics as a competitive and often glory- or money-seeking venture. In addition, athletes and their sponsors have often looked to nutritional intake for quick and easy answers. In the past people experimented with such varying practices as fluid restriction, laxatives, vegetarian diets, fasting, even bloodletting. And within recent times athletes have turned to large vitamin doses, protein tablets, and drugs.

Athletes in the United States today have lost the spirit of the ancient Greeks. We have become a nation interested in specialized sports, mostly on a professional level, and when we or our children indulge in athletics, it is usually on a highly competitive basis rather than for personal growth and health. However, one advantage of competitive sports is that organized and big-business-oriented athletics have fostered some interest in research into nutritional benefits. Nevertheless, the limited amount of information available is generally in very esoteric form and appears in journals that never reach the average American.

Naturally, nutrition guidance should begin in the prena-

tal period. The unborn child's potential for good health is
dependent upon many factors, including the quality of his
parents' seed, the state of the mother's health during pregnancy, and the mother's diet during pregnancy. Subsequently
the child is dependent on his parents not only to provide good
nutrition for the first few years of life, but to instill a knowledge of and respect for proper diet throughout life.

Every man, woman, and child in the country should involve themselves to some degree in some form of sport for
their own health. We can't all be top Olympic athletes, but we
can evaluate our personal capacities, body type, age, and
physical restrictions (congenital or acquired), and by following proper nutrition attitudes we can operate at optimal levels.

In *Nutrition and the Athlete* we have synthesized all
available information on diet and nutrition relating to sports
and exercise. Naturally, before one begins to apply nutritional information to athletic performance, one must be aware
of what nutrition is. Therefore, the early part of this book is
devoted to an explanation of foods and diet. We also provide
specific information concerning nutrition for children, teenagers, and women. Only after understanding nutrition can the
reader appreciate the application of nutrition and diet to training and participation in athletic activities.

2 FOODS AND NUTRITION

All people have some knowledge of their own body. To what degree depends entirely on the interest level of the individual. It is important at this point to explore within the given limitations of this book the factors contributing to the health of the body in relation to athletic performance.

The motivation and energy expenditure of the body have both physiological and psychological components. The scope of this book deals primarily with the physiological aspects. We do, however, investigate the psychological nature of sports in later chapters.

The human body is an extraordinarily efficient energy-conversion apparatus. (We define energy, in this case, as the capacity to do work.) Energy exists in two forms: *kinetic energy* is an active form of energy such as motion, heat, light, and electricity; *potential energy* is chemical energy that the body transforms into kinetic energy, as when food is turned into heat and movement.

The measuring unit for expressing the energy content of food is the *large calorie*, or *kilocalorie*, which can be defined as the amount of energy needed to raise 1 kilogram (2.2 lbs.) of water 1 degree centigrade. Therefore, if a given amount of food containing 400 calories was burned and the heat transferred to 1 kilogram of water, the temperature of the water would rise by 400°C.

METABOLISM

The energy requirements of the human body are high. Metabolism of the body is defined as all of the chemical reactions that require energy. Metabolism involves two reactions: those in which food is broken down and energy is released, and those in which new substances are produced within the body and energy is stored up.

The essential activities of the body (such as heartbeat, breathing, and glandular secretions) demand energy. This energy expenditure for ordinary body functioning is called the *basal metabolic rate* (BMR). The BMR is different for every person, varying by degrees for several reasons and in several instances.

- Relative size differences. Women usually have a lower BMR than men.

- Periods of growth. The BMR rises during the first five years of life, levels off, rises again just before and during puberty, and then declines into old age.

- Size of the individual. Smaller bodies tend to have a higher BMR.

- Fever generally raises the BMR approximately 7 percent for each 1°F rise.

- Minor BMR differences occur among different races; for example, the BMR of some Orientals is lower than that of Caucasians.

- In most cases the BMR rises in response to lower temperatures as a compensation mechanism to maintain body temperature.

- The BMR rises during lactation, because milk production utilizes energy. This is a large increase (about 60 percent, or 1,000 calories) because breast milk has a value of 30 calories per ounce, and the average daily production is about 30 ounces.

- Pregnancy raises the BMR.

- Thyroxine stimulates the BMR.

- Starvation and malnutrition lower the BMR.

- Diseases increase the BMR.

On the average a full-grown adult uses 1,500 to 1,800 calories per day for his BMR. People can calculate the number of calories necessary per day to maintain their own BMRs by multiplying 24 calories (one for every hour of the day) by the number of kilograms (2.2 pounds) of body weight.

The range of energy needs extends from about the number required for BMR to more than twice that amount, depending on the degree of activity of the body in question.

ENERGY AND CALORIE CONSUMPTION

If varying sums of energy are spent in varying ways, it is reasonable to say that there will be varying caloric requirements. To illustrate, swimming the crawl requires 14 calories per minute, whereas volleyball requires around 3½ calories per minute. In order to maintain optimum performance level and optimum functioning weight most athletes during active periods require between 3,500 and 6,500 calories per day. A relatively inactive person may use as few as 500 additional calories per day.

Muscular contraction requires the change of chemical energy into mechanical energy. The chemical energy comes from a combustion process—the oxidation (or burning) of nutrients, proteins, carbohydrates, or fats. It is a well-established fact that muscular energy resulting from energy transformation is proportional to oxygen consumption. In other words, the food we eat is changed by the body into energy to perform all of its functions.

A report of the 1973 meeting of the Food and Agriculture Organization on Nutrition in Rome states that

> The energy requirements of individuals depend upon four variables interrelated in a complex way: (a) physical activity, (b) body size and composition, (c) age, and (d) climate and other ecological factors. . . . Individuals of the same size living in the same environment and with the same mode of life have a similar energy requirement whatever their ethnic origin. . . . Among individuals of the same sex and body size and age, the amount of physical activity is usually the most important factor causing variations in energy expenditure.

Where do we get all of this energy? From food, of course. Not only is food the source of physical and mental energy for the body, it is also used for

Raw material for building and maintaining tissues
Body heat
Insulation
Tissue accumulation
Sustaining normal blood sugar level
Sustaining normal acid-base balance
Body fluids
Controlling substances (such as vitamins and minerals)
Storing energy
Hunger satisfaction
Appetite satisfaction

We may define nutrition as a process that begins with the ingestion of food and ends with the functioning of the body. Inasmuch as sports activity requires more energy than is necessary for a daily living routine, a larger amount of food must be consumed by athletes. Our definition of sports is used in the very widest sense to mean any athletic activity, from professional football to weekend jogging.

Calorie Needs

All people must vary their own food intake according to the amount of physical energy expended. It stands to reason that a professional football player must take in greater amounts of food than a sedentary elderly person whose activity consists of walks in the park on Sundays.

During the preliminary period of athletic activity—in the form of a regular organized training program—the caloric intake fluctuates according to the specific needs for gaining or losing weight. If the individual is to attain a satisfactory weight, caloric intake must balance the output. If this balance is not maintained, the results will range from underweight—causing lassitude, general inefficiency, and lack of stamina—to overweight—causing impediment of muscular activity and fat overload, which ultimately may be fatal.

Different athletic undertakings "burn" varying amounts of calories, depending on the energy demands placed on the body by the stress of the activity. Table 2.1 lists a number of common foods and their calorie content, including how much time is needed to utilize those calories by specific activities. Table 2.2 indicates energy expenditure per hour during different exercises for a person weighing approximately 154 pounds.

Types of Energy

It should be understood that energy is not created; it exists in varying forms that are endlessly being transformed from one to the other by the process of metabolism. The infinite cycle of energy has the sun as its ultimate source of power. Through a system called photosynthesis, which utilizes carbon dioxide and water as raw materials, plants change the sun's energy into food storage forms. The body in turn takes these nutrients (chemical energy) and "burns" them to release other forms of energy in the body, including *electrical energy*, as in nerve and brain activity; *thermal energy*, as in regulation of body temperature; *mechanical*

TABLE 2.1
CALORIES IN COMMON FOODS, AND ACTIVITY TIMES NEEDED TO UTILIZE THEM

FOOD	CALORIES	ACTIVITY				
		Walking*	Riding bicycle†	Swimming‡	Running#	Reclining‖
		min.	min.	min.	min.	min.
Apple, large	101	19	12	9	5	78
Bacon, 2 strips	96	18	12	9	5	74
Banana, small	88	17	11	8	4	68
Beans, green, 1 c.	27	5	3	2	1	21
Beer, 1 glass	114	22	14	10	6	88
Bread and butter	78	15	10	7	4	60
Cake, 1/12, 2-layer	356	68	43	32	18	274
Carbonated beverage, 1 glass	106	20	13	9	5	82
Carrot, raw	42	8	5	4	2	32
Cereal, dry, ½ c., with milk and sugar	200	38	24	18	10	154
Cheese, cottage, 1 Tbsp.	27	5	3	2	1	21
Cheese, Cheddar, 1 oz.	111	21	14	10	6	85
Chicken, fried, ½ breast	232	45	28	21	12	178
Chicken, "TV" dinner	542	104	66	48	28	417
Cookie, plain, 148/lb.	15	3	2	1	1	12
Cookie, chocolate chip	51	10	6	5	3	39
Doughnut	151	29	18	13	8	116
Egg, fried	110	21	13	10	6	85
Egg, boiled	77	15	9	7	4	59
French dressing, 1 Tbsp.	59	11	7	5	3	45
Halibut steak, ¼ lb.	205	39	25	18	11	158
Ham, 2 slices	167	32	20	15	9	128
Ice cream, 1/6 qt.	193	37	24	17	10	148
Ice cream soda	255	49	31	23	13	196

Food	Calories	Walking*	Riding bicycle†	Swimming‡	Running#	Reclining¶
Ice milk, 1/6 qt.	144	28	18	13	7	111
Gelatin, with cream	117	23	14	10	6	90
Malted milk shake	502	97	61	45	26	386
Mayonnaise, 1 Tbsp.	92	18	11	8	5	71
Milk, 1 glass	166	32	20	15	9	128
Milk, skim, 1 glass	81	16	10	7	4	62
Milk shake	421	81	51	38	22	324
Orange, medium	68	13	8	6	4	52
Orange juice, 1 glass	120	23	15	11	6	92
Pancake with sirup	124	24	15	11	6	95
Peach, medium	46	9	6	4	2	35
Peas, green, ½ c.	56	11	7	5	3	43
Pie, apple, 1/6	377	73	46	34	19	290
Pie, raisin, 1/6	437	84	53	39	23	336
Pizza, cheese, ⅛	180	35	22	16	9	138
Pork chop, loin	314	60	38	28	16	242
Potato chips, 1 serving	108	21	13	10	6	83
Sandwiches						
Club	590	113	72	53	30	454
Hamburger	350	67	43	31	18	269
Roast beef with gravy	430	83	52	38	22	331
Tuna fish salad	278	53	34	25	14	214
Sherbet, 1/6 qt.	177	34	22	16	9	136
Shrimp, French fried	180	35	22	16	9	138
Spaghetti, 1 serving	396	76	48	35	20	305
Steak, T-bone	235	45	29	21	12	181
Strawberry shortcake	400	77	49	36	21	308

*Energy cost of walking for 70-kg. individual = 5.2 calories per minute at 3.5 m.p.h.
†Energy cost of riding bicycle = 8.2 calories per minute.
‡Energy cost of swimming = 11.2 calories per minute.
#Energy cost of running = 19.4 calories per minute.
¶Energy cost of reclining = 1.3 calories per minute.
From Frank Konishi, "Food Energy Equivalents of Various Activities. *Journal of the American Dietetic Association* 46 (1965), pp. 186–188.

TABLE 2.2
ENERGY EXPENDED PER HOUR BY 154-POUND PERSON
IN VARIOUS PHYSICAL ACTIVITIES

ACTIVITY	CALORIES PER HOUR
light exercise	170
walking slowly (2.6 mph)	200
active exercise	290
severe exercise	450
swimming	500
running (5.3 mph)	570
very severe exercise	600
walking very fast (5.3 mph)	650
walking upstairs	1,110

energy, as in the contraction of muscles; and varying types of *chemical energy,* as in the production of new compounds (hormones, and so on).

No matter what form of energy is used the reservoir of "free" energy is tapped. Consequently the system must be replenished constantly, and in the case of the human body, this source is food.

DIGESTION

It is not enough simply to ingest adequate food for energy. Another important consideration is the *absorption* of food, or the conversion of food substances into body substances. This transformation is done by mechanical and chemical means that break down the ingested food into particles small enough to be absorbed by the body. The absorption process begins with chewing (mastication), a process that combines the food with saliva, making it easier to swallow and more acceptable by the stomach. An enzyme released with the saliva, *ptyalin,* begins breaking down the starch molecule even before it enters the stomach.

The liquids and partially softened foods then enter the stomach to be acted upon by gastric juices (stomach acids) for further breakdown. From the stomach the food passes rather quickly into the small intestine by the peristaltic contractions of the stomach. Different foods leave the stomach at different rates—fats more slowly than proteins, proteins more slowly than carbohydrates.

It is in the small intestine that secretions from the gall bladder, pancreas, liver, and intestinal mucosa act on the food. It is here that the most crucial processes of digestion occur, which result in the fundamental substances of food being absorbed into the bloodstream and assimilated by body tissues. Substances such as bile and vitamins accelerate the absorption of fats and other nutrients into the bloodstream.

In the case of liquid food, however, there is little digestive activity in the small intestine. There are many advantages to a liquid meal over a solid meal in preparation for sports. We discuss this aspect in Chapter 6.

The large intestine has little to do with actual digestion except that it permits rapid absorption of fluids, which are necessary for digestive processes. As is the case in all fuel utilization there is a certain amount of residue, and in the body this is excreted within 12 to 24 hours.

As we mentioned earlier, the metabolic rate and efficiency of the body functions vary from individual to individual. Therefore, it is necessary to alter nutrient intake to compensate for this inefficiency factor, and to maximize the absorption of nutrients to obtain maximum energy output. There are five factors most conducive to maximum digestion: gastrointestinal motility, neural and hormonal regulators, sufficient digestive enzymes, appetizing and palatable foods, and an anxiety-free environment.

We don't have direct control over those conditions that are dependent on genetic patterns, such as gastrointestinal motility and neural and hormonal regulators. However, we can control the rest. In the case of appetizing and palatable foods and an anxiety-free environment the ways to success are obvious, but as for sufficient digestive enzymes the answer is a bit more complex. We feel that with an athlete's occasional excessively high intake of protein, for example, it would be advantageous to supplement the diet with digestive enzymes in the form of oral tablets. This addition would not only maximize efficient absorption, but it would eliminate the sometimes attendant distress of gas forming as a result of incomplete digestion. One should not put an excess load of food on the system without aiding it, if possible.

There is, however, a restriction of digestant intake, specifically hydrochloric acid (HCL), by those who suffer from ulcers. In this case one should seek the assistance of a physician knowledgeable in nutrition.

THREE FOOD COMPONENTS

Let us now examine the component factors of food and how they work in the body. Even with all the external dissimilarity among the hundreds of kinds of food eaten by people, they can still all be classified into three categories: carbohydrates (C), fats (F), and proteins (P), or any combination of the three. Each of these is considered as important as the others, and so the quality of diet is based fundamentally on a balance of these components, rather than on an imbalanced intake of any one of them.

In spite of almost universal lip service to this basic truth, theories contrary to it flourish. Of course, in terms of sports and diet some of these theories do have some short-term validity. For example, a pregame meal should have a greater carbohydrate than fat or protein content, and during training periods individuals may have a higher protein intake. These varied food intakes can be rationalized for short periods only, however; essentially, the premise of balance should be adhered to.

It is important for everyone, but especially athletes, to

know as much as possible about food. Thus, we include this abbreviated description of the three basic food groups.

Carbohydrates

Carbohydrates are composed of starches and sugars and are the most important energy sources available. They are complex organic compounds made up of the elements carbon, hydrogen, and oxygen. There are three important types of carbohydrates present in food—polysaccharides, disaccharides, and monosaccharides.

Polysaccharides are complex carbohydrates called starches, which are long molecular chains of simple sugar units linked together. The polysaccharide cellulose, which is the fibrous residue of plant tissue after digestion, cannot be transformed into energy by man for lack of an enzyme to assist in its breakdown. But because of its structure it adds bulk, or roughage, to the diet, stimulating the lower intestinal tract for optimal functioning and formation of the feces. If the intestinal tract is not cleansed properly, it may accumulate putrefactive waste, decreasing the efficiency of the body and thereby detracting from maximum athletic performance.

Disaccharides consist of two simple sugars. Examples of disaccharides are sucrose, or common table sugar (cane and beet sugars being identical); maltose, made by germinating grains; and lactose, found only in milk.

Monosaccharides are units of simple sugar, either glucose (a form of dextrose) or fructose (fruit sugar); the most important of these is glucose. Most of the carbohydrates used by the body—whether in the form of mono-, di-, or polysaccharides—are converted eventually into glucose during the process of digestion and at the beginning of metabolism.

Although glucose is the major source of energy, some of it is turned into fat and stored in the adipose (thick, fatty) tissue for possible future use. Other carbohydrates combine with other elements to form more complex molecules.

Each pound of carbohydrate eaten yields 1,860 calories of energy. Even if the food intake is low in carbohydrates, the body will convert fats and protein into glucose to provide energy. Table 2.3 compares the energy values of the basic food groups.

Throughout history, of all the basic nutrients that sustain man, carbohydrates have been of prime importance for essentially four reasons.

1. Availability. Carbohydrates make up most of the world's food supply. They are contained in such easily grown plants as vegetables, grains, and fruits. In some countries carbohydrates make up almost the entire diet of the population. Even in relatively wealthy countries, such as America, where many food sources are available, about half of the total caloric intake is comprised of carbohydrates.

2. Storage ease. By comparison, such carbohydrate foods as grains, and some fruits and vegetables, can be kept in dry storage without spoilage for extended periods of time. Advanced packaging and processing have further extended the storage life of some carbohydrate foods almost indefinitely. Meat and dairy products, on the other hand, require controlled conditions such as refrigeration for storage.

3. Low cost. It reasonably follows that due to the accessibility and wide distribution of carbohydrates, the

TABLE 2.3
CALORIES IN THE THREE FOOD GROUPS

TYPE OF FOOD	CALORIES PER GRAM	CALORIES PER POUND
Carbohydrate	4.1	1,860
Protein	4.1	1,860
Fats	9.3	4,220

cost is comparatively low. It has been shown that when the economy of an individual, group, or nation declines, the proportion of carbohydrate intake increases. On the other hand, protein foods are the most expensive.

4. Energy value. Because of the easily available glucose equivalent of carbohydrates, man relies on them as his prime fuel source.

The amount of carbohydrates stored in the body is relatively small. A total of approximately 365 grams is stored in muscle tissue and the liver and present in circulating blood sugars. Following is the distribution of carbohydrate in a person weighing approximately 154 pounds:

liver glycogen	110 grams
muscle glycogen	245 grams
extracellular blood sugar	10 grams
total	365 grams, which equals an energy output of 1,460 calories.

These 365 grams of carbohydrates provide enough energy to maintain bodily functions for about 13 hours. In order to meet this energy demand, then, carbohydrates must be eaten regularly and frequently.

Three factors contribute to the way in which carbohydrates are used by the body.

1. Endocrine functioning, especially insulin and insulin antagonist. Irregularity and inefficiency among the various hormones greatly affect the body's use of carbohydrate.

2. The condition of the mucous membrane of the digestive tract and the health of the bowel lining.

3. Vitamins, which must be available in sufficient amounts to metabolize carbohydrates. The B-complex

vitamins are especially necessary to perform key
functions in the enzyme systems for carbohydrate
oxidation.

Carbohydrates also serve special purposes in vital organs. In the liver, for example, they are oxidized as fuel, and
in the form of glycogen they also detoxify toxic materials
such as drugs. The resulting harmless substance is subsequently excreted. Carbohydrates also have a controlling influence on fat and protein metabolism. In other words, the presence of carbohydrates allows the protein to be used for its
basic structural purpose of tissue building and repair.

Healthy heart contractions are a fundamental prerequisite for worthwhile athletic activity. Glycogen in the heart is
an important emergency origin of contractile energy. If a
heart is in disrepair, an inadequate carbohydrate intake may
cause cardiac symptoms, or angina. The central nervous system depends on a steady supply of carbohydrate for proper
functioning. Because the brain (the body's regulating center)
contains no facilities for glucose storage, it depends on the
glucose in the blood supply (blood sugar). Irreversible brain
damage may occur as a result of insufficient carbohydrates
being supplied to the brain.

The chief function of glucose is to supply energy according to the individual demand. This supply of energy is controlled by hormone activity, which raises or lowers the blood
sugar. An oversupply creates a condition called diabetes, and
an undersupply creates the opposite condition called hypo-
glycemia, or low blood sugar. Insulin is the hormone produced
by the body that controls oversupplies of blood sugar, and
glucagon raises the blood sugar level.

Fats

Fats are defined as a group of organic substances—oils,
fats, waxes, and related compounds—that are greasy to the
touch and insoluble in water. The so-called visible fats are
margarine and butter, oils and salad dressings, bacon and
cream. The so-called invisible fats are egg yolk, meat fats,

olives, avocado, and nut meats. Fat yields 4,220 calories per pound, which is over twice as many as carbohydrates. Fats therefore have the highest energy content of any foods. They also provide a reservoir of energy for long-term storage. The fat reservoirs are found under the skin, around ovaries and kidneys, and interspersed with the muscles. In the case of food restriction the subcutanous fat responds first and is most adaptable.

In addition to its function as an energy storehouse, fat provides essential unsaturated fatty acids along with palatability, aroma, and flavor. Besides this absorption of fat-soluble vitamins and fat is important in the membranes of every cell and in nerve sheaths. When the stores of carbohydrates are utilized, the body breaks down tissue fat and protein to provide additional energy. It is important to the athlete to have an adequate amount of fat in the diet to prevent the breakdown of body protein, which is needed for tissue reconstruction.

There have been no limits to the amount of fat a body can store up when the caloric intake exceeds energy expenditure. In most cases the energy output of the athlete generally offsets an inordinate amount of fats ingested, but as athletic endeavors diminish and the fat intake does not, obesity develops. This syndrome should be carefully watched, especially as the athlete grows older and less active.

The proportion of fat in the daily caloric intake for the average person in Canada and the United States ranges from 35 to 44 percent. This is high in relation to carbohydrate and protein intake. The range of athletes, considering their added activity, should be from only 20 to 35 percent. Even though fat provides more energy than do proteins or carbohydrates, it releases the energy more slowly, and thereby endurance is impaired. Carbohydrates are the preferred nutrients for quick and prolonged energy expenditures. In athletics that involve minimal energy expenditure mixed with rest periods, diets dominant in fat or carbohydrates do equally well. For athletics of a strenuous nature, unrelieved by rest periods, carbohydrates are best, according to Jean Mayer in an article entitled "Food Fads for Athletes" in the *Atlantic Monthly*, December 1961.

Fats lend palatability to food. Actually, most people require its presence to make the meal acceptable. Also, meals with high fat content are high in satisfaction because they stay in the stomach longer, because of the slow absorption rate.

Fatty acids are the basic components of fats, and they may be saturated or unsaturated. A saturated fatty acid has all available bonds of its molecules filled with hydrogen. The more saturated fat is, the harder or more solid it is. Butter and lard are examples of saturated fats. Unsaturated fats, which are free-flowing and liquid at room temperature, are usually of plant origin. Vegetable oils are unsaturated fats.

The term *essential* when applied to fatty acid refers, first, to whether its absence will create a specific deficiency disease (for instance, a certain eczema is caused as a result of no linoleic acid—unsaturated fatty acid—in the diet), and second, to the fact that if the body cannot manufacture it, it therefore must be obtained from the diet.

There are three polyunsaturated fatty acids—linoleic, linolenic, and arachidonic. These are called essential simply because they are necessary for normal life. These three fatty acids perform the following functions in the body:

- They fortify capillary and cell membrane structure.

- They combine with cholesterol to form cholesterol esters, thereby enabling the body to handle the cholesterol easily.

- They lower serum cholesterol.

- They prolong blood-clotting time to aid in healing.

Another important aspect of fat is its structural function, which is to pad vital organs against impact and to hold them in place. In addition, the subcutanous layer of fat provides

insulation against heat and cold. Thus, fat is not only important from a chemical point of view, it is also necessary for
protection in rough contact sports activities such as football,
soccer, and boxing.

Cholesterol is manufactured by the body from fats and
is related essentially to the sex and adrenal hormones. High
cholesterol counts generally become impeding and often fatal
by clogging the arteries and inhibiting blood flow. Diminishing the intake of cholesterol foods such as eggs, dairy products, and refined carbohydrates, along with supplementation
of lecithin (a phospholipide that disperses cholesterol in the
arteries), is generally suggested to reduce this count.

The digestion of fats takes place only in the small intestine, although the initial preparation for fat digestion occurs
earlier, in parts of the gastrointestinal tract. The fats in the
small intestine are acted upon by chemical agents from the
gall bladder, liver, pancreas, and the small intestine itself, and
are broken down by enzymatic action. The remaining fat is
secreted into the large intestine and subsequently eliminated
as fecal fat.

Inasmuch as fat and carbohydrate metabolism are so
interrelated, the same hormones that affect carbohydrate metabolism also affect fat metabolism. There are three of these
hormones:

1. Growth hormone (GH), adrenocorticotrophic hormone
   (ACTH), and thyroid-stimulating hormone (TSH) are
   all secreted by the pituitary gland, which increases
   the release of free fatty acids from adipose tissue by
   imposing energy demands on the body.

2. The adrenal gland releases cortisone and hydrocortisone, which causes the release of free fatty acids.

3. Thyroxine, a hormone secreted by the thyroid gland,
   stimulates the release of free fatty acids from adipose
   tissue and lowers blood cholesterol.

There has not been any optimum allowance established for fat intake for support of maximum health. Each individual must take the responsibility to maintain that all-important balance of foods from each food group. This, combined with proper weight maintenence and sufficient exercise, will allow the body to correct itself according to its biological individuality.

Protein

Proteins are organic substances that, after digestion, yield their component building blocks—amino acids. Proteins are found in animal foods, such as milk, meat, eggs, and cheese, and to a lesser extent in plant foods, such as grains and legumes. The highest quality protein is found in egg white. This is said to have a high biologic value, since the protein contains all eight essential amino acids. A protein low in one or more of the essential amino acids is said to be of low biologic value. These eight amino acids are essential in that the body needs them for normal growth and development, yet is unable to manufacture them. The other amino acids are nonessential, since the body can manufacture them when required to do so.

Most proteins from animal sources are of high biologic value, while proteins from plant sources are of low biologic value. In fundamental terms it is not the amount of protein one ingests that is important, but the quality of protein.

Proteins are further classed as complete or incomplete. Complete proteins contain all of the essential amino acids in adequate quantities and balance to supply the body's needs. These proteins are meat, eggs, milk, and cheese. Incomplete proteins are deficient in one or more essential amino acids and are of plant origin—legumes, nuts, and grains. In a balanced diet the animal and plant proteins supplement one another. In many cases incomplete protein sources can be combined to form complete proteins—for instance, alfalfa sprouts and peanut butter together provide all the essential amino acids. This point should be well heeded by vegetarians, who usually receive insufficient amounts of complete proteins.

The fundamental function of protein is the maintenance and growth of tissue. It also contributes to the body's muscle energy metabolism. Estimates claim that an average of 58 percent of the total dietary protein becomes available as glucose and is utilized to yield energy.

The symptoms of protein deficiency are varied and rather nonspecific. Immature symptoms are lassitude, loss of weight, easy fatigability, diminished resistance to disease, prolonged convalescence, and, in children, slow stunted growth. Advanced protein deprivation results in low blood protein levels, edema, and liver damage.

Requirements for protein seem to vary according to the source. The Food and Nutrition Board of the National Research Council suggests one gram of protein for every kilogram (2.2 pounds) of body weight. This means that a person weighing 70 kilograms (154 pounds) should ingest 70 grams of protein per day. Other nutritional authorities such as Adelle Davis have claimed that in light of current ecological stress and muscular development needed for athletics, the intake should be one gram of protein for every pound of body weight. Individuals can perhaps calculate their own intake requirements by gauging how different amounts of protein affect their performance, general feeling, and health. The Food and Nutrition Board also suggests 78 grams per day for pregnant females and 98 grams per day during lactation periods. By comparison to Canadian standards, U.S. standards here are generous.

It has been shown that protein is not metabolized in significant amounts during muscular exercise in the well-nourished person. Consequently, it need be considered only briefly as having any quick-energy action. Exercising does not significantly increase the protein requirement.

Coaches and athletes have traditionally stressed the need for eating lots of meat. The general belief is that athletic activity causes a loss of muscle protein, which can be replenished by eating meat. This theory has been generally refuted by many authorities, but the practice continues, perhaps as more of a psychological motivation. In fact, the protein requirements of the body are determined by the rate of growth, not by athletic activity. Seemingly, the only persons requiring greater amounts of protein are high school athletes and those who are interested in increasing muscle mass, such as bodybuilders and weightlifters.

FOOD SUPPLEMENTS

Now that we have discussed the three major food groups, we can consider food supplements, both vitamin and mineral. There has been and will undoubtedly continue to be controversy on supplementing the normal diet from food sources with manufactured vitamins and minerals.

Vitamins

Although vitamins are neither body-building nor energy-giving, they are essential in varying quantities as links in the metabolism of other nutrients in the maintenance of physiologic well-being. These organic compounds cannot be synthesized by the body, and so must be replenished regularly. This survey approaches vitamins only to the extent of their importance in relation to athletic activity. The reader may look to other sources for a more comprehensive study.

Vitamins are found in varying amounts in different foods. No one food contains all the vitamins necessary for optimal growth and body maintenance. Unlike carbohydrates, proteins, and fats, vitamins are necessary in relatively small amounts. This can be explained by the fact that vitamins are catalytic in nature—they simply "spark" the efficiency, mobilization, and assimilation of other nutrients.

Classically, vitamins are divided into two major groups: First, the *water-soluble vitamins*, C and B-complex, require water presence for their absorption into the body, and they are lost through urination. They are not stored in the body to any appreciable degree, and so a constant dietary supply is necessary to avoid their depletion and the resulting impediment of physiologic functioning. Second, the *fat-soluble vitamins*, A, D, E, and K, require the presence of dietary fats for absorption. They are not lost in urination and tend to store in the body. A day-to-day supply is thus not required for maximum functioning.

The complete absence of any given vitamin from a diet creates a condition called *avitaminosis*. A diet that falls below the minimum requirements of one or more vitamins yields a condition known as *hypovitaminosis*. Such a diet does not create any serious illness, but it does detract from health and vitality, thereby preventing the enjoyment of a full life. We believe that the stresses placed on persons involved in exercises, coupled with the fact that most people suffer from subclinical deficiencies, makes supplementation necessary. The application of vitamins to athletics is used throughout the book according to the scope of the individual chapters.

Vitamin E

There has been a great deal of current controversy on the effects of vitamin E on athletic performance.

Recently, investigators have studied whether vitamin E can maximize energy output and thus aid athletes in increasing performance. In animal experimentation muscular dystrophy has resulted from vitamin E deficiency. This type of testing has raised the question of whether or not the excessive strain sports place on the muscular system may mean that the requirements should be higher for athletes than for those on an ordinary diet. Another study showed that vitamin E assisted in lung control of oxygen in experimental animals.

This particular aspect gained prominence at the Olympic Games at Mexico City in 1968, where the high altitude adversely affected long-distance runners.

Several reports claim that vitamin E can improve performance. In a series of studies T. K. Cureton found that

giving athletes doses of vitamin E benefited their performance. In a more recent study, reported in the Los Angeles
Times of September 20, 1974, Dr. Lester Packer found that
human lung cells, which normally die after reproducing themselves 50 times, reproduced themselves 120 times with vitamin E. Although vitamin E did not reverse other aging processes in the human body, Dr. Packer concluded that it
"might prevent an early death, or brain disease, heart attacks, or senility."

These findings bear obvious significance to athletes, who
are constantly searching for ways to improve their cardiovascular systems to increase endurance.

In relation to air pollution Dr. Packer says, ". . . the
ability of a cell to survive depends on its capacity to correct
or eliminate the buildup of environmental pollutants, and by
providing these cells with vitamin E we may be able to tip the
scales in favor of the cell's survival in this environment."

He continues by explaining his belief that human cell
death is not predetermined, but is influenced by environmental pollution such as nitrogen dioxide, ozone, and excessive
molecular oxygen.

While the conclusions about vitamin E therapy have been
generally favorable, there have not been scientific and statis-
tical grounds for empirical verification. We feel, however,
that supplementation of this vitamin will prove beneficial to
physical performance. The richest sources of vitamin E are
the vegetable oils (unrefined), unrefined cereal products (especially wheat germ), and eggs. Of the oils, crude wheat germ
oil contains the highest amount of vitamin E; soybean oil is
next.

Minerals

Minerals are absorbed by the body as simple compounds.
Once they are in the body, however, they are used in complex
ways. Many minerals are necessary for optimal nutrition.
They are interrelated with each other to perform particular
body functions. Some minerals—calcium, for instance—are

TABLE 2.4

FUNCTIONS AND SOURCES OF KEY NUTRIENTS

NUTRIENTS	FUNCTION	MAJOR SOURCES
Calcium	Helps build bones and teeth; helps blood clot; helps muscles and nerves react normally; helps tired muscles recover and delays fatigue.	Milk, cheese, ice cream; turnip and mustard greens, collards, kale, broccoli
Iron	Combines with protein to make hemoglobin, the red substance in blood that carries oxygen to cells.	Meat (especially liver), eggs, dried beans, green leafy vegetables, some dried fruits like raisins and prunes.
Iodine	Makes thyroxine, an essential hormone that regulates metabolic rate. Prevents (simple) goiter.	Seafoods, iodized salt.
Phosphorus	Helps build bones and teeth and to regulate many internal activities of the body.	Liver, fish, poultry, eggs, cheese, milk, whole-grain cereals, nuts.
Protein	Builds and repairs all tissues; helps form antibodies to fight infection; supplies energy.	Meat, fish, poultry, eggs, cheese, milk, dried beans and peas, peanut butter.

TABLE 2.4 (con't)

NUTRIENTS	FUNCTION	MAJOR SOURCES
Fat	Supplies large amount of energy in small amount of food; helps keep skin healthy by supplying essential fatty acids	Butter and cream, whole milk, salad oils and dressings, cooking fats, fat meats
Carbohydrate (sugar and starches)	Supplies energy; carries other nutrients present in foods.	Bread and cereals, potatoes and corn, dried and sweetened fruits, sugar, jelly, syrup, honey
Vitamin A	Helps keep skin clear and smooth; helps keep mucous membranes healthy and resistant to infection; helps prevent night blindness; helps control bone growth	Liver, deep yellow fruits, dark green and yellow vegetables, butter, cream, ice cream, whole milk, yellow cheese.
Thiamine (vitamin B1)	Helps promote normal appetite and digestion; helps keep nervous system healthy and prevent irritability; helps body release energy from food	All meats (especially pork), fish, poultry, eggs, enriched and whole-grain breads and cereals, milk, white potatoes
Riboflavin	Helps cells use oxygen; helps keep vision clear; helps keep skin and tongue smooth; prevents scaly, greasy skin around mouth and nose.	Milk, cheese, ice cream, meats (especially liver), fish, poultry, eggs

TABLE 2.4 (con't)

NUTRIENTS	FUNCTION	MAJOR SOURCES
Niacin	Helps keep nervous system healthy; helps keep skin, mouth, tongue, digestive tract in healthy condition; helps cells use other nutrients.	Peanut butter, meat, fish, poultry, milk (high in tryptophan), enriched or whole-grain bread and cereals
Vitamin B6, Vitamin B12, and Folacin	Helps prevent anemia; helps enzyme and other biochemical systems function normally	Vitamin B6: meats, potatoes, dark green leafy vegetables, whole grains and dry beans; vitamin B12: milk, cheese, eggs, and meats; folocin: green vegetables, whole grains, and dry beans
Ascorbic Acid (Vitamin C)	Helps to make cementing materials that hold cells together; strengthens walls of blood vessels; helps resist infection; helps prevent fatigue; helps heal wounds and broken bones.	Citrus fruits, strawberries, cantaloupes, tomatoes; broccoli, green peppers, raw cabbage, white potatoes
Vitamin D	Helps the body absorb calcium from the digestive tract and build calcium and phosphorus into bones	Vitamin D milk, fish-liver oils, sunshine on skin
Vitamin K	Maintains normal clotting functions of the blood	Pork liver and yolk of egg, green leafy vegetables, lettuce, cauliflower

directly related to the development of healthy bones and teeth, and others aid in the hormone production. Calcium is also utilized by the body to regulate the heartbeat and to exert a balance between potassium and sodium in maintaining muscle tone.

Impaired muscle action and coordination and hyperirritability are sometimes consequences of low blood calcium levels. Under normal circumstances calcium catalyzes the change of chemical energy into meaningful muscular contractions, according to *Nutritional Data,* a compendium of nutritional information published in 1962 by the H. J. Heinz Co. The remaining essential minerals, which are considered rarely lacking in the American diet, are sodium, potassium, chlorine, copper, sulphur, zinc, manganese, and magnesium.

The amounts of supplementation are instituted by the individuality of the athlete. Table 2.4 lists the food constituents and their sources. By self-observation and performance trial-and-error the athlete may be able to determine his own needs. If this poses a problem, a nutritional physician can assist.

3 NUTRITIONAL CONDITIONING THROUGH THE YEARS

Nutritional conditioning commences the moment one is conceived, but nutritional changes are incorporated as the body changes from infancy to childhood, from adolescence to adulthood. Naturally, growing children have specific needs, as do teenagers. Adult women's needs differ from those of adult men.

PROGRAMS FOR YOUTH

The Youth Fitness Council was initiated during the Eisenhower administration and revitalized and vigorously promoted during the Kennedy administration. The Council sponsored a survey in five states among 200,000 children, grades 4 to 12, to determine the facts concerning youth fitness. Less than 10 percent of those in the survey had reached a satisfactory level of physical performance. Physical education consumed less than two hours per week, while TV watching ranged from 15 to 30 hours per week. Only 28 percent of the schools studied had adequate health and physical education programs, and 50 percent did not have a daily program. To make the picture even bleaker, it was found that 25 percent of the youths were overweight, and that physical activity is geared by the schools for those who need it least of all, the athletes, who constitute a mere 10 percent of the total.

The council moved to improve this dismal picture. First, they prepared guidelines for schools on health education, physical education, and nutrition. Nineteen educational and medical organizations assisted in preparing these guides.

Several basic principles were outlined as essential for an effective physical fitness program, including vigorous activity, progressive resistance exercises, and maximum nutrition. They also mentioned that for the development of muscular strength activity should be more than 50 percent of strength capacity; that organ efficiency is enhanced by physical activity over a long unbroken period; and that the degrees of endurance and power are the essential components of physical fitness.

Because a great deal of children's time is spent in school, it is important that there be proper assignment and preparation of teachers to strengthen the health education programs.

Particular emphasis is placed on the elementary school, where the fundamentals of athletic and dietary patterns are formed. There should be continued evaluation of physical education, which should be graded just like any other subject in the curriculum. The council's manual also provides guides for teaching load, class size, and teaching stations. There is also an emphasis on physical education as a basic experience that should not be replaced by activities such as athletics or ROTC. The manual emphasizes the importance of intramural sports for children in grades 4 to 12, overseen by competent leadership. Particular importance is placed on teams, leagues, tournament, play days, and demonstrations. Not only the gifted, but all should have the opportunity to participate in intramural activity. There should be special concern placed on the development and maintenance of clubs in such areas as cycling, hiking, camping, and skating, along with provisions for informal play and activity.

Social agencies outside the school system should complement physical education programs by bringing these activities beyond the classroom and into the community. Special emphasis is placed on the role of colleges and universities as centers for research and education, serving as guides through in-service training and physical development and research.

We feel that the council has done a great deal to stimulate the ideals of proper exercise and nutrition to aid in the development of children into normal adulthood.

BABIES AND TODDLERS

The best years for building an excellent body, attitudes, and patterns are between birth and age three. It is generally during these years that people becomes whatever they are going to be. There are many ideas contrary to this, but a case can be made for comparing a child to anything that is built— a piece of furniture, for example, is only a fine piece when its components are fine; their being that way is the reason for its ending that way. No matter how people are subsequently educated or trained, they are simply logical extensions of those first three years.

The attitudes of the parents are essentially the attitudes of their offspring. We feel it is the moral responsibility of the parents to ensure proper dietary habits. Breast feeding is the healthiest and most rewarding form of infant nutrition. Children fed this way, it has been shown by Carlton Fredericks and other authorities, develop more satisfactorily during this entire period.

Research has shown that the required amount of vitamin D administered to babies was not enough to protect them against rickets. It was discovered that breast-fed babies receive an enzyme called phosphatase that lowers the vitamin D requirements, whereas babies fed cow's milk did not. It appears that the pasteurization process destroys this enzyme. Breast feeding is far and away the best method of infant nutrition.

Growth Patterns

Children grow at their own pace. Let the child do it naturally. This individuality expresses itself in food and activity, likes and dislikes, rest and attitudes toward people and peers. It is important to allow the child to develop individually within the framework of the parents' love and understanding and an intelligent attitude toward healthful food, activity, peaceful rest, and discipline that can be understood.

Often parents in their overzealous enthusiasm for the proper growth of the infant become anxious if the child does not meet certain growth standards that the standard charts predict. This concern is unfounded. What is important is that the child *grows*. There are periods in child development where growth is retarded somewhat. This is no cause for alarm, even though the child may have a smaller appetite and become less active. Again, this is normal in most cases and should be viewed calmly.

The parents should see to it that the child is examined by a physician once every six months during the first six years, to ensure that development is progressing normally and to deter as much illness as possible.

Activities

The activity of the infant and child before the age of five depends on the parents. Some parents make a point of allowing their children to experience as much as possible of their environment, by allowing free crawling and investigation—of course, within the limits of safety. Some intelligent and aware parents we know of show their infants everything possible. They carry their babies to various objects such as plants, trees, paintings, furniture—anything that holds interest. This allows the children to develop curiosity and, in turn, develops their interest in the world and encourages a healthy acceptance of the environment.

As far as exercise is concerned, the parent should allow free movement within the given confines of a playpen or similar area. The most elaborate scheme we have heard of is parents padding an entire room halfway up the wall, filling it with playthings both creative and amusing, and allowing the child free domain in the room. This allows the child sufficient exercise to maintain maximum growth rate. Even though this type of scheme is not within the reach of most people, it is possible to modify this setup to suit every family situation.

Feeding

Another basic interest to develop in children is a fundamental enjoyment of food. This can be done by feeding them in pleasant and agreeable surroundings and by offering as broad a spectrum of food as possible. Many times a child develops certain likes or dislikes as a result of the parents making a fuss over certain foods. This can be eliminated simply by not taking any attitude toward particular foods. Try to offer all foods with approximately equal enthusiasm. Children are individual enough without the parents inflicting their attitudes on them.

The infant usually receives adequate amounts of vitamins D and C from mother's milk. If this is not the case, a vitamin D supplement should be given. If the baby is being fed cow's milk, a vitamin C formula should be given in the form of drops. There are many commercial preparations on the market, and a physician should be able to recommend one. A source of iron should be added to the infant diet, too, although this addition is not necessary if the formula is iron fortified.

As the infant becomes older, the addition of solid foods is essential, usually between one month and three months. The quality of commercially prepared baby foods is higher than parent-prepared foods for three reasons. First, baby-food producers generally maintain their processing plants near the source of food, which means that it is more likely to be fresher than food the parent can purchase. Second, these commercial food processing companies design their systems to retain the maximum amounts of nutrients, whereas the parent cannot ensure this technique in the household. Third, less than 1 percent of fresh produce is inspected for insecticide residues, thus creating a potential health hazard. The commercial processor must maintain rigorous contamination controls, thereby obtaining the purest foods possible.

A point to be remembered is that many commercially prepared baby foods contain sugar, which is unnecessary and which raises the infants' vitamin requirements without satisfying them. In this formative period of lifelong eating habits it is wise not to condition the taste buds to too much sugar. Thus, there should be a gradual addition of foods such as egg yolk, strained meat, and fish. When the child is old enough to express desires, the addition of sweets to the diet should be made on a sound nutritional basis. Commercial candy should never be given to children; suggested substitutes include homemade pastries low in sugar or homemade candies made with fruits. Iced confections can be made with unsweetened frozen juices.

An inexpensive, sound supplement to a baby's diet is wheat germ. (Many commercial preparations contain it, too.) A fraction of a teaspoon of wheat germ can be added to cereal. Remember that it is necessary to pulverize the wheat germ to avoid any mechanical irritation to the baby's digestive tract.

The addition of more solid foods should be instituted as soon as possible—but not prematurely. If such food is introduced too soon, the unselective digestive tract might form allergies. Conversely, the sooner strained meat is included, the greater will be the growth and development of the body, along with an increased resistance to infection. Additional nutritional insurance is available in the form of small amounts of brewers' yeast, which contains essential B vitamins.

Since most children develop certain likes and dislikes in food, it is sensible to include a vitamin-mineral supplement in the diet to ensure adequate nutrition. There are many well-balanced commercial supplements available, and one needs simply to employ intelligent selection in purchasing. If problems arise, a pediatrician will surely direct the parent properly.

PRESCHOOL CHILDREN

Older preschool children grow less rapidly than one- or two-year-olds, but they are more active. They need foods with energy and growth qualities. The diet should contain larger portions of meat, fish, eggs, as well as plenty of fruit and vegetables, whole milk, and whole-grain cereals and bread. American children receive much less vitamin A than necessary, so it is important to include dark-green and yellow vegetables such as broccoli, collards, kale, carrots, sweet potatoes, and winter squash. Butter also provides vitamin A.

This age group requires high amounts of vitamin C, too, which may call for a vitamin C supplement. A liquid preparation supplying 100 milligrams of vitamin C per day is sufficient for this group.

Most preschool children like snacks. This is recommended, but the parents must ensure that the snacks are nutritious as well as tasty. The snack should not be oversweetened; whole-grain cookies or crackers fortified with wheat germ are excellent. Children like protein snacks—ham, cheese, hard-boiled eggs, or crackers with cottage cheese or peanut butter are nutritious.

The preschool activity ratio is high and should be encouraged. Often games that children play greatly enhance muscular coordination and development. The need for practice allows them to keep up and going. Allow safe opportunities to run, climb, and explore. The more a child exercises, the easier the job of feeding will be, thereby allowing the parents to pick and choose wisely. The most powerful force in learning is imitation; if the parents eat properly, chances are the children will also.

Some children grow fat because they are taught to eat more than necessary. Their habits are dictated by the socioeconomic environment of the parents rather than the food needs of the child. It is advisable to serve small amounts of food and allow the child to come back for seconds. The habit of overeating usually continues on into adulthood, with all of the attendant disadvantages of obesity.

CHILDREN IN ELEMENTARY SCHOOL

As children progress to school age, their activity rate is even greater, and diet demands are therefore increased. It is important at this time for the parents to establish some sort of routine—tailored within limits to the individual likes and dislikes of the child, of course, rather than to those of the parents. It seems that when an orderly pattern of playtime, naptime, mealtime, and bedtime is adhered to, the child develops better both physically and emotionally.

Many parents set a structure on a child's eating time. Apparently as soon as the keen edge is taken off the child's hunger, time is of no importance, and some dawdling may occur. Rushing the child will only serve to discourage the pleasure of eating. There are situations when time is important, and in those cases an explanation should be offered to the older child, while the younger child should be helped along.

Children may go on food jags, too, wanting a certain food every day for a long stretch and then suddenly switching to demand another food. If it is not too impractical, the parents should be casual about this. Experience has proven that giving in to a child's whims and being reasonable and less demanding eventually results in the child's being more reasonable and less demanding himself.

Do not make too many rules for the child. They only serve to confuse. A few direct simple rules give the parent a grasp on development and the child's emotional security. Do not demand that the plate be completely clean before dessert; give small portions and allow for seconds. If the child sits and plays with the food, remove it quietly without fuss or threats. The next time the child will think more clearly and then remember.

BODY TYPES

As children grow they enter one of the three major body build divisions set up by the physiologists:

Ectomorph—the thinnish nervous type
Mesomorph—mostly athletic, muscular, bony type
Endomorph—overweight, tending toward obesity

These types serve mainly as a warning to the parent to avoid the extremes. The contributing factors that develop these types are essentially genetic inheritance and nutrition. The tall, thin person has the opportunity to become a top athletic runner or a scarecrow. Mesomorphic children who are denied exercise and proper diet may very well become endomorphs.

Essentially speaking, if one parent is fat, a child has a 40 percent chance of being fat also. Of course, if both parents are fat, the percentage is increased. If the basics of development—proper nutrition, rest, and exercise—are applied to children, it is possible to modify the inherited build. It is of course true that certain builds are suited to particular athletic pursuits. If the parents provide the proper environment early in life, they mold a happy, fulfilled child. If they ignore a child, the potential is limited and it serves to create an unhappy child.

If the ectomorphs have the talent along with the attention needed to develop skills, they may very well develop into top runners or tennis players. This does not imply that other athletic fields are closed to this type of individual, it just means that upon careful observation those who are most successful at these endeavors are generally of this type.

When given the opportunity, mesomorphs usually become skilled at contact sports. Endomorphs are of course rather limited in their choices. However, most fat children are not fated to be that way if carefully supervised. Many fat children have both grace and flexibility, and if given the proper exercise and diet, they can easily participate on an equal footing with their peers. It is up to the parents to take stock of their children and see which way they tend. Then appropriate steps can be taken.

A child who has been raised with proper nutrition and exercise will never be fat or fatigued. Too many people refer to a fat child with such euphemisms as chubby, baby fat, adolescent fat. These divisions are all just plain fat.

In many instances children raised on a diet loaded with fats and carbohydrates grow fat before they can control it themselves. When children are fed and cared for properly, their skin is clear, teeth beautiful, hair shiny, eyes bright, and body slender, straight, and alert. Children who are fat, tired, and pimply are often simply showing the effects of an inadequate diet. Parents should eliminate junk foods such as sweets, soda pop, potato chips, cakes, and gum.

Nourishment simply must be adequate to support the extra stress of children's attempts to comprehend their environment and their considerable physical exertion. The nutritional planning for children up to the age of 12 generally depends on such factors as geography, climate, and historical, sociological, technological, and economic differences.

TEENAGERS

Between the ages of 12 and 18 certain biological changes occur. Along with these changes there is a corresponding differentiation in the performance curves of boys and girls. In both sexes there occurs an increase in daily nutritional needs, which is especially important to the teenage athlete of both sexes.

Boys
The first thing to do is determine the body build the boy has inherited. This can be done by examining the parents,

aunts, and uncles. The goal is to strive for optimum development within the individual framework.

The four basic rules for maximum health and development are:

1. Desire for physical activity
2. Rest and relaxation
3. Regular exercise
4. Good nutrition

Since we are dealing with primarily nutrition, we shall expand on that. A growing teenage boy has food requirements that are higher than at any other time. The reason for this is rapid development and growth along with increased athletic activity. The well-nourished adolescent boy will be more alert and enthusiastic, ready to do more things, in addition to being more confident as a result of his fine appearance. Sound nutrition allows the body to build up reserve energy that can be used for more work and extra recreational activities.

The five main determinates of food needs are:

1. Growth—during adolescence growth is at its maximum, and so proper food is important to ensure proper development of organs, muscles, and bones.

2. Physical activity—a full schedule of sports, work, school, and social activities creates a great demand upon the diet.

3. Size—if one is taller than average, more nutrients are needed to maintain that size.

4. Special needs—overweight, underweight, or other conditions.

5. General appearance—condition of skin, hair, eyes, gums, and teeth are influenced by diet.

Calories are an important consideration in food selection. Boys need more calories, generally speaking, than girls because of size differentiation. Even though calories are a consideration, nutrients should be considered as primary, since it is easier to get calories. The boy should accumulate calories in the form of good food rather than junk foods, which add bulk but no nourishment. The following data will help in computing how many calories a boy needs. Remember that this is an approximation and that no two boys are alike.

TABLE 3.1
THE CALORIE NEEDS OF BOYS

AGE	9–12	12–15	15–18
calories per pound per day	33	31	25

Thus, a boy 9–12 years old who weighs 72 pounds should take in about 2,400 calories per day. A boy 12–15 who weighs 98 pounds needs about 3,000 calories per day, and a boy 15–18 and 134 pounds needs about 3,400 calories per day.

What a boy eats during the day is important. Foods from each food group should be ingested daily, incorporating three meals a day plus sensible snacks. The following is a framework meal plan that can be used as a guide. This sample menu will provide approximately 1,600 to 2,200 calories, according to the foods selected.

Breakfast is probably the most important meal for the teenage boy. The time from the last meal at night to breakfast is the longest span, and the highly active teenage boy needs to resupply the energy lost during that period. A good, nutritious breakfast ensures a good supply of energy throughout the day, with a decrease in the fatigue factor that generally occurs during school in the midmorning slump. A good breakfast also ensures that postathletic activities will be charged with the greatest amount of energy application.

In many cases there is a problem of overweight, often because the height of the body has not caught up to its weight. If this is the case, there is little cause for alarm. If the heavy weight is determined to be detrimental, then a decrease in high-calorie foods and an increase in protein-rich foods is necessary until the appropriate weight is achieved. A boy is often overweight because he has eaten too many overly rich foods such as pies, ice cream, candy, and soda. These foods provide high calories with little of the other nutrients that contribute to maximum bodily efficiency.

Increased physical activity also helps in weight reduction as well as in toning the muscles that may lose tone as a result of weight loss. When losing weight, try not to lose more than a pound per week. The reader is referred to the training and weight section for a detailed account of this concept (see Chapter 4).

Many times the weight problem of the teenage body is one of underweight. This may develop as a result of too little sleep, or if not enough time is devoted to substantial meals made up of the right foods.

Weight should not be gained at more than one pound per week. During this time extra physical activity will ensure that the weight gained is muscle and strong tissue, not fat. This is the time to create a strong healthy body for the future as a healthy adult.

Desiccated liver tablets and yeast tablets, along with a well-balanced vitamin-mineral supplement, are vital substances needed for growth. Because of the denatured state of contemporary food, it is often difficult to procure the proper nutrients without these additions.

Girls

The teenage period is one of rapid growth for girls, and special attention must be paid to the demands of sports during this period.

Because of the psychological changes a female undergoes during these years, the good food habits acquired during childhood are often cast aside temporarily. The teenage girl is apt to acquire irregular food habits, skipping breakfast or lunch and eating more junk foods, which contain only empty calories, devoid of other nutrients. This type of eating detracts greatly from the functioning efficiency necessary for various athletic pursuits. A good appetite is sometimes simply not enough to guarantee proper nutritional habits. When she satisfies hunger with empty calories, the teenage female athlete may be contributing to some retarded organ or muscular development that may in time prove irreversibly damaging.

The teenage girl sometimes avoids eating for fear of gaining too much weight, even though there is no apparent problem with obesity. Her diet is generally selected by her peer group rather than her parents or someone who is knowledgeable. On the other hand, some teenage girls develop a pattern of overeating that is difficult to break in later life.

Because of the loss of iron in the blood during menstrual flow, the chances of a female developing anemia are greater than with males. Thus, such iron-rich foods as liver and dark-green, leafy vegetables should be generously included in her diet. If the diet is well supplied with these foods and an anemic condition persists, supplementation with iron tablets and desiccated liver tablets should be considered.

Breakfast should include a generous portion of milk along with 2 or 3 ounces of animal protein (egg, ham, or sausage) in addition to a whole-grain cereal or bread. As has been mentioned, a skimpy breakfast usually leads to a slump later in the day. This can only result in decreased athletic performance. An adequate breakfast will also discourage snacking of junk foods later in the day.

The teenage girl should have at least four servings daily from the vegetable-fruit group. Apples, bananas, oranges, and grapefruit should be eaten in season. Along with the citrus fruits, raw tomatoes provide vitamin C. In addition, servings of dark-green or deep-yellow vegetables or fruits should be eaten daily. Greens, broccoli, spinach, sweet potatoes, squash, carrots, cantaloupes, and peaches provide a rich supply of vitamin A.

The breads and grains should be whole grains and whole-grain products. Processed, bleached flour and flour products are devoid of vital nutrients and supply empty carbohydrates that add weight without nutrient value. Three slices per day of rich, whole-grain, dark bread or ½ to ¾ cup of whole grain cereals (the granola cereals are especially good) provide the necessary nutrients from this food group.

It has always amazed us that people haven't realized that whole-grain bread and other products are not only superior in nutrient value, but are also superior in taste value! No one can convince us that a lifeless slice of processed, bleached white bread is nearly as appetizing as a rich, whole-grain one. Only social conditioning has led us to believe otherwise. Experiment for yourself, and remember that the closer to nature the food is, the higher is its nutritional value.

In cooking vegetables and fruits, the rawer the better. Vegetables should be steamed for a short period to ensure maximum food value. When cooked in this manner, they should be a bit hard to the bite. The Italians have a marvelous expression to describe this consistency—*al dente*, literally translated, "to the teeth," or simply a bit undercooked.

The meat group—meat, fish, poultry, eggs, and cheese; as alternatives, beans, peas, nuts, and nut butters—should be supplied at least twice a day.

Snacks are important and often necessary. Because the teenage female athlete expends a great deal of energy and is also in a rapid-growth period, the standard diet is often not enough. A great many snack foods come into play, and it is our belief that they can be beneficial. Instead of lifeless potato chips, candy, and sugared soft drinks, substitute such foods as mixtures of sunflower seeds, raw nuts, and raisins. This combination fills the need for food and something sweet, but also provides extra calories in the form of protein and fructose (fruit sugar). Fresh fruit juices, which are far more satisfying in nutrition and in taste, should be substituted for worthless sugared soft drinks.

Healthful foods are generally more appealing than destructive foods. We feel that snacks of this sort will only supplement an already complete diet, which in turn will provide maximum nutrients for the teenage female athlete to carry on her activities efficiently. Sugar, candies, syrup, jellies, soft drinks, and alcohol add calories, but few nutrients, to the diet. When counting calories, not only is the amount important, but the quality is, too. Fruit juices supply vitamin C as well as a midday pickup; soft drinks provide nothing more than calories. A plate of fresh fruit for dessert, instead of apple pie, provides vitamins C and A in addition to calories.

Many tests have been conducted on body weight in relation to diet and energy expenditure, with results published in the various and numerous medical journals. The following, we feel, bears direct significance on our subject. In the August 1973 issue of the *Archives of Environemental Health* a test was outlined to display the cardiorespiratory responses of young overweight women to energy expenditure following modest weight reduction.

Twenty-four overweight women participated in this 15-week program. They were divided into three groups according to weight-reduction regimens: diet; exercise; and combined diet and exercise. The diet allowed for a 500-calorie-per-day reduction, and the exercise consisted of intermittent walking and jogging, or just one of the two, three to five days per week. The results showed that diet and exercise were equally effective in producing modest but significant loss in body weight over the 15 weeks. But the subjects who participated in diet and regular exercise not only lost weight, they also improved the cardiorespiratory fitness level.

THE SPECIAL NEEDS OF WOMEN

The physiological differences between men and women are significant. We have included the two areas that are relevant only to the female—pregnancy and menopause. It is our feeling that these two stress situations should receive special attention concerning their relationship to athletics. When the female attends to the proper physical and psychological needs during these periods, she will maintain exuberant good health through them.

It seems that women are more concerned with their weight than men generally are. This may be a significant factor in the findings that Americans lead the world in death from coronary heart disease (CHD) with the greatest increases among men in their thirties, forties, and fifties. One factor that eliminates a great deal of CHD among women is the immunizing effect of the female hormone, estrogen, which was used at one time as therapy by injecting it into males who had suffered heart attacks. The amount of estrogen required for maximum protection was so high, however, that some secondary female sex characteristics began to develop in the patients.

The presence of this hormone in the female begins to decline as menopause occurs. The decrease in the hormone causes an increase of the risk of heart attacks among women. This fact, coupled with the added stress of jobs that were one time male jobs, makes for a great deal of stress on the mature female. It is important, then, for women to be concerned with exercise and diet to prevent a mass increase in CHD.

Physically, females develop before males until puberty. They become capable of sexual reproduction between the ages of 12 and 14. During the puberty years males develop larger, heavier bones, additional body weight, and greater muscle mass. During this period females develop fat deposits that create the rounded, soft body contours that are generally associated with feminine sex appeal. Because of her wider hips and the slightly different angle of the thighbone as set in the hip socket, the female's walk and carriage are different from the male's. This swaying movement as opposed to the straight male movement affects the athletic capacity.

Researchers and observers have noted that males reach their maximum natural fitness during their late teens and early twenties; females, on the other hand, reach their peaks during puberty and the middle teens. There is a steady fitness decline from these ages on, unless it is maintained through proper exercise and diet.

Changing Standards in Athletics

At one time athletic females were considered to be masculine, and their physical activities would raise many controversial remarks. Happily, things are changing, mainly as a result of the women's liberation movement in this country. Most people are coming to realize that exercise does not build unattractive muscles in the female, and that female athletes are as attractive and feminine as females with other interests.

Because of contemporary females' newfound interest in athletics, it is worthwhile to devote a special section to their particular problems and needs.

Prior to the time of the Greeks, there is hardly any evidence of any organized athletics for females. The Babylonian Code of Hammurabi, however, specified that "all people" should participate in exercises. Great minds throughout history have ordained that women should participate in sports. Plato felt that in the ideal state men and women should have the same sort of gymnastics training. In the complex Greek city-state of Sparta the women trained in the public square under the supervision of female trainers.

From the fall of Rome to the Renaissance women did not participate in sports to any great extent. This was largely because strong overtones of asceticism and scholasticism coupled with distorted medieval concepts of chivalry were particularly unfavorable to female athletic activity. During the enlightened period of the Renaissance women began once again to share an almost equal footing with men in athletics. However, the fundamental female activity was still care of the house and child rearing. Certain athletic endeavors became known as feminine and were therefore acceptable. These activities of the seventeenth century included handball, club ball, and archery. Later on, specific movements included women in their organizational plans.

It was not until 1899, at the Conference on Physical Training, that the U.S. first recognized women in sports by appointing a committee to make an extensive study of modifying the rules of basketball so that it could be played by women. It was this committee that first published "girls' rules" for the sport. Essentially, these rules stressed standards to ensure the health and welfare of the participants according to the prevailing standards of the day.

This "breakthrough" committee set a trend that was subsequently followed by similar rule modifications in soccer, track and field, swimming, and hockey. It also set in motion the events that led to the formation of a Committee on Women's Athletics in 1917, by Dr. William Burdick and the American Physical Education Association. All these committees and movements were finally combined in 1932 by the foundation of the National Section of Women's Athletics.

Most of the committees for women's sports were founded on pseudobiological evidence differentiating between women and men. Most of these concepts were founded, of course, on the prevailing sociophilosophical traditions of the society. The biological differences have, as mentioned earlier in this book, some bearing on restricting activity. However, these differences of height, weight, organic structure, body type, inhalation, metabolism, and endocrine secretions are restrictive to males, too.

It is due to the dynamic influence of people such as Gloria Steinem and Germaine Greer along with such influential female athletes as Billie Jean King that the current attitude of the society is changing. The customs of our society are changing rapidly to allow all women to participate in sports with enthusiasm and vigor equal to that of the male.

Probably the most important topic in regard to female activity in sports is the menstrual period. It was thought that women must be guarded against any physical or emotional stress during this time. However, it is now understood that reasonable physical exercise during menstruation is not only allowed, but encouraged, especially for women who experience painful menstruation (dysmenorrhea). Exercise improves circulation, muscular strength, and flexibility in the abdominal region, which relieves the discomforts of cramps and lower backache. Conditioning strengthens the body against the monthly stress. It has been demonstrated that many outstanding Olympic performances occurred during the menstrual period of the athlete. In the case of heavy first day blood flow, however, it is suggested that a woman refrain from competition.

It was during the twenties in America that the really objective research was carried out on sex differences. There was a great deal of data to support the view that some differences are justifiably related to sex. Once these differences are brought into the proper perspective, however, they lose their significance in terms of function and behavior. It is this understanding that fosters an intelligent pattern of athletics for women.

Ultimately, then, athletics should be participated in by all women from 6 to 60, according to each individual's physiology and psychology. All women cannot be track and field stars, nor do they want to be, but every woman can at least take long walks, jog, bicycle, hike, and engage in other healthful physical activities. Athletics for females will continue to survive and maintain an equal position with male athletics without the masculine overtones of the past as long as they are participated in, directed by, and needed by women.

There are some other physical considerations involved, such as the breasts. A great many women are under the impression that exercise will increase the breast size excessively. This is untrue; what exercise does is normalize the breast. If the breasts are too small, exercise will increase their size; if the breasts are too large, exercise will decrease their size. Of course, if specific breast-building exercises are performed, the development is controlled by the individual. This normalization effect takes place over the entire body, ensuring the maximum degree of development for that given individual's potential.

Differences Between the Sexes

When considering the anatomical differences between males and females, we must begin with the skeletal differences. From birth, certain bones in the metacarpals and phalanges of the female ossify before those in the male. The knee joint of the female is more stable for its size than that of the male because of its wider construction. The female has less bone mass than the male, and the length of the adult male bone is greater. According to authorities the increased size and weight of the male muscle pulling and stretching the bones may well account for their increased size. These same authorities conclude that generally the male has a more prominent nose, a squarer jaw, higher cheekbones, heavier ends of the long bones, and deeper grooves where the muscles attach.

With her narrower shoulders and wider hips the female's arm may have a different angle from that of the male. The universality of skeletal anatomy between the sexes is evident, but generally the female bony pelvis is broader and shallower than that of the male. Coupled with the adipose tissue padding over the hips, the female hips appear exaggerated.

The entire growth pattern of the female is faster than that of the male. It has been estimated that girls achieve growth 2.24 years before boys. However, as far as adult height is concerned, the average female is 5 to 6 inches shorter than the male. In weight the male is 20 to 25 percent heavier than the female. There is a variance in the average center of gravity between male and female. The female's is about 0.6 percent lower than that of the male, a difference that is created mainly by males' greater height, broader shoulders, and narrower hips.

Certain anatomical differences create advantages and disadvantages for both male and female. For example, the lower leg of the female may be shorter than that of the male, and generally the male foot is greater in length and width than the female's. The man's arm is generally longer. The male's longer development period produces a more massive, heavier person with certain structural advantages, especially in the upper body. Of course, we are speaking in broad terms, and these differences vary from individual to individual. The quality of a given performance in a given sport is determined by the anatomy of the individual, not by the gender of that person.

Along with the anatomical differences, there are certain functional differences to consider. The prime difference may be the larger heart of the male, brought upon by a greater muscle mass needing more circulation. This size difference creates a higher heartbeat rate in females.

Physiologists have estimated that the mean red blood corpuscle count in the male is 5 million per cubic millimeter compared with 4 million per cubic millimeter in the female. The male blood has approximately 8 percent more hemoglobin, and the specific gravity of male blood is higher than female. Finally, both the diastolic and systolic pressures are generally about 5 to 10 percent higher in the male.

Because of the female's smaller thoracic cavity and smaller lungs there is a tendency toward respiratory acceleration. Thus, the breathing capacity is lowered.

The metabolic rate is higher in the male at all ages than in the female. This rate is changed to a minor degree in the female during the periodic sexual cycle, and allegedly this influences the red blood corpuscle count, the respiration rate, hemoglobin count, and blood's specific gravity. There is some speculation that the female's lower metabolic rate is caused by the presence of excess adipose tissue in relation to protoplasmic tissue. There is also a theory that the metabolic rate is related to sex differentiation and thus may be a cause and/ or effect of sex determination.

In the female there is a faster calcium metabolism rate assumed to be the result of earlier ossification of the bones. On the other hand, the larger and more massive male bone structure indicates that calcium retention is greater in the male.

Although generally speaking the muscle mass of the female is less than that of the male, there is no indication that athletic muscular coordination is any less in the female than in the male. It is of course true that the greater the muscle mass, the greater the strength, but strength is not necessarily equated with gender. Some observations have shown that the reaction time is quicker in boys than in girls from 6 to 17, but no further indication claims that this speed persists into adult-hood.

To summarize this discussion of physical development, we repeat that exercise and sports do not make the female figure unattractive. On the contrary, every normal girl needs exercise to train the muscles to respond gracefully and readily to the conscious or unconscious directions of the individual. Exercise is a normal, rewarding way to develop grace in movement and in posture. It is simply a harmonious working together of the structural parts of the body. This development will result in coordination and rhythm as opposed to wasteful effort and awkwardness.

Pregnancy

Pregnancy is a legitimate reason for alteration of exercise, although not one for its omission. The nervous fatigue often associated with pregnancy is decreased by exercise. Most knowledgeable obstetricians insist that their patients exercise during pregnancy. In addition, there is reason to believe that exercise and proper diet prior to conception eliminate chronic fatigue, which may be a factor affecting the normal menstrual flow and thus disrupts the ovulatory pattern.

The age span that is the most active for childbearing is

from 20 to 40. Thus, if a woman is going to carry the extra weight of pregnancy, it is important that she condition the muscles and tissue to withstand the extra stress. The women of certain primitive tribes sometimes give birth in the morning and return to the fields in the afternoon to resume normal work. This results from top conditioning, which can only be maintained through sound diet and exercise.

Diet is especially important during pregnancy. For example, if at particular times during gestation there is a nutritional deficiency, abnormalities in the fetus may occur. It is important to have a proper diet when the organs and structures are first being formed. It has long been known that innate deformities are often caused by malnutrition. Deficiencies of vitamin A, riboflavin, folic acid, pantothenic acid, B12, and vitamin E have caused such structural abnormalities as deformed eyes, brain malfunction, heart malfunction, aorta defects, kidney defects, genito-urinary abnormalities, cleft palate, harelip, extra toes, and hernia of the diaphragm.

There have been many experiments designed to see whether improved diets can produce healthier babies. An example of this would be a study made by Guttorm Toverud of Oslo, Norway. Using supernutrition over a period of six years, he found stillbirths to be decreased by half. Premature births and infant mortality within the first month were also reduced by half, while brain hemorrhages and bone-deficiency conditions like rickets practically disappeared. The common ailments of pregnancy such as leg cramps, anemia, numbness in the fingers and toes, neurologic pains, constipation, high blood pressure, and excess water retention were also all curtailed as a result of improved nutrition. The very important ability to breast feed was also improved.

Of course, tests of this sort usually have dramatic effects due to the close, controlled nutritional supervision. Although few people are generally under these conditions, it is surely the moral responsibility of the individual to maintain maximum nutrition before and during pregnancy.

An experiment at the University of Pennsylvania Medical

School divided a group of expectant mothers into two groups: one was given a vitamin supplement along with nutritional instruction, and the other did not receive instruction and vitamin supplementation was left to their own discretion. In the first group there were fewer than a dozen premature births, while with the other group the incidence of prematurities was 5 percent, the American national average percentage. In the instructed group the incidence of prematurity was 80 percent lower than the national rate.

Varicose veins during pregnancy are said to stem from several different causes. Some say that a lack of exercise allows the muscle to lose its tone and a vein its elasticity. Therefore, the blood doesn't circulate properly. If this is the case, specialized exercise to improve circulation and muscle tone will remedy the condition. Others say the problem is more chemical than mechanical. Dr. William Coda Martin, in an article in the *Western Journal of Surgery, Obstetrics, and Gynecology* (Vol. 50, 1942) claimed that women who were supplied with generous amounts of vitamin C during pregnancy were much less susceptible to varicosities. According to Dr. Martin the problem arises as a result of nutritional deficiencies that create undue stress on the veins, rather than from the added weight of pregnancy creating the strain.

Another chemical theory is that during pregnancy the production of female hormone is high, and that this hormone affects the veins. A well-balanced diet will help the mother to keep this hormone activity in check. Our feeling is that both exercise and diet cover all possibilities, so it would be wise to ensure the proper addition of both.

Pregnancy diets should begin at least six months to one year before conception. This allows the body time to recover from any deficiency it may have suffered. Pregnant women should eat the same amount of food as before, with emphasis on a higher protein intake and less fats and carbohydrates. Proteins are basic for the mother's body maintenance and necessary for proper growth and development of the fetus. In addition, protein is used by the body to ensure good lactation.

Certain obstetricians advise a higher intake of protein foods such as meat, egg, fish, and poultry.

Sugar intake should be limited. Carlton Fredericks, Roger Williams, and others have pointed to evidence that strongly indicates excessive sugar intake to be responsible for such problems as hardening of the arteries, difficult menstrual cycle, varicosities, and complications of pregnancy.

The B vitamins are the antistress vitamins. In addition, inadequate supplies of these vitamins for a woman during pregnancy may result in her baby having a lower IQ than the average. It has also been noted that when pregnancy nausea persists, an addition of vitamin B6 to a vitamin B-complex syrup administered to the mother will generally correct this condition.

The expectant mother should have at least one quart of milk per day. This prevents calcium loss and ensures enough calcium and vitamin D for healthy development of the baby's bones and teeth. Along with this, eggs and generous servings of meat, fish, or poultry should be included in the diet. Iron-rich foods such as liver, heart, kidney, shellfish, and egg yolks should be eaten often. The pregnant female also needs generous amounts of citrus fruits, tomatoes, deep-yellow and green leafy vegetables daily. There should be less emphasis on rice, noodles, fried or greasy foods, fats, breads, and sweets. Physicians often prescribe vitamin supplements such as vitamin D and C in addition to a proper diet. Pastries, ice cream, nuts, and candy should be avoided as much as possible.

It is wise to remember that pregnancy is not the time to correct the nutritional mistakes of an entire lifetime. Any woman asking this from a diet is certainly naive. The time to start one's improved nutrition is the present, from infancy on.

Menopause

Menopause is indeed an exclusively female problem. There are many women who live in fear of this period in life. It should be clearly noted, first, that menopause is indeed inevitable, and second, that there are certain steps to take to decrease the disadvantages of this period.

Exercise should by all means be continued through the menopause. Demonstrations have shown that because of the decrease of the female hormone, estrogen, there is a decrease in the body's immunizing substances. This clearly indicates that the maintenance of strong muscle and tissue will ensure maximum defense against maladies if and when they occur. Also, as one's age advances, the chance of elective-type surgery increases, and postoperative complications are decreased if the woman is fit. Exercise will also impart esthetic qualities to the body and give a psychological lift.

Unfortunately, the stresses of modern-day society inflict terrible anxieties on the menopausal woman. She is often given sedatives for nervousness or irritability and female hormones for their altering effect. These conditions can be attenuated somewhat through a regular exercise program.

The tranquilizers may have a decided long-term negative effect (see Chapter 7 on drugs), and the synthetic hormones may give rise to a risk of cancer formation. The truth is that the nutritional information and sources available to modern women can alter the magnitude of the menopause experience.

The theory behind the administration of the synthetic female hormones is that when they occur naturally, there are disturbances in the change of life. This is much more severe when menopause is induced by hysterectomy.

An article in the *Journal of the American Medical Association* "Gynecology—A Surgical Necessity or Therapeutic Racket?" reported that 400 sets of organs removed in a series of 1,100 hysterectomies were discovered to be normal; if proper examination procedures had been applied, surgery could have been avoided. The fact is that Americans are overfed and undernourished. The major reason for hysterectomies, fibroid tumors, can be controlled and eliminated by the application of sound nutritional rules. These principles will ensure the most comfortable time during menopause.

Vitamin E is effective therapy during menopause. There is a great deal of research using this vitamin, and interested readers would do well in conducting research into this themselves. Vitamin E has quieted anxieties, decreased irritability, and in many cases totally eliminated unnecessary perspiration and heat sensations. If adequate supplies had been given throughout the life of the individual, the chances are that aging would have been much less arduous.

The B-complex vitamins in combination with calcium produce a calming, quieting effect upon an ordinarily jumpy menopausal woman. When these factors are added to a diet high in protein, medium in fat, and low in carbohydrate, the woman will usually respond to a satisfactory degree, thereby eliminating the need for tranquilizers, sedation, and female hormone therapy. The menopausal woman must remember that eating habits that have been developed over the years are difficult to overcome. It is usually these patterns—which were decided and developed when the body was in a different state—that cause obesity when carried into menopause. So, in order to eliminate overweight, diet alterations must be an important consideration for the menopausal woman.

Finally, the psychological trauma of menopause also can be reduced if the woman is prepared with a fit body as a result of nutrition and exercise.

FEEDING ADULT ATHLETES

Sound nutritional feeding of the athlete is essentially no different from feeding an ordinary citizen. An adequate diet to maintain energy and dexterity is essential not only on days of a game, but every day. It is important to maintain conditioning on a long-term basis.

It is true that the energy needs of an athlete are considerably higher than those of more sedentary persons—depending on the sport and the degree of participation of each person. Logically, a professional ball player has much greater demands placed on the body than a middle-aged weekend jogger. Anyone involved in physical activity should consume enough nutrients to balance energy expenditure and to maintain normal body weight and maximum efficiency. Each individual differs in the exact amount of food needed for this, but body weights usually indicate to what extent the diet works.

Records of body weight should be maintained on a weekly or monthly basis. The weight chart in this book on p. 83 serves as a skeletal indicator; the athletes themselves or their coaches usually know which weights are most desirable for any activity. Allowing athletes to select their own diets may lead to their not having enough stamina to maintain the activity. Admittedly, nutrition is not the sole factor in determining a poor or a good performance, but those who look at it irresponsibly may carry unnecessary impediments.

The best time for educating athletes in nutrition is when they are highly motivated to improve their performances. It is up to the athletic integrity of both the coach and the athletes to accept the nutritional knowledge presented to them.

Athletes must strive to maintain proper dietary habits as part of their lives. This will ensure maximum efficiency throughout life. In an article in *Preventive Medicine* (1972, pp. 409–421) the following is cited:

> . . . analysis has shown that certain common habits of daily life, called good health habits, are positively related to physical health status. Further, the relationship of these habits was shown to be cumulative; those who reported all or many of the good practices were in better physical health, even though older, than those who followed fewer such habits.

We know that nutritional deficiencies impair performance. What we are primarily concerned with here is what can be done through diet to increase the efficiency of those who are not clearly underfed or malnourished.

Muscular activity increases not only the body's caloric requirements but also its need for the B vitamins, which work in the enzyme systems that are fundamental to energy exchange. When sweating creates losses of sodium chloride, it must be regained.

Sports activity creates a general increase in the consumption of all ordinary types of foods, including milk, butter, meat, fish, eggs, and cheese. The athlete must not let a monotonous diet increase the risk of a deficiency in unknown or poorly known nutrients or of losing the motivation to continue good eating.

Ordinarily, the salting of foods is adequate to provide the salt needed for sports activity. Many times, however, cramps attributed to salt deficiency have been reported in high-energy contact sports such as football. This situation has been relieved by the addition of bouillon cubes to the diet.

Sedentary people require as much protein as very active people, but they need less fat and carbohydrates. This can be explained by the fact that protein simply supplies the building blocks for growth, whereas the energy comes from fats and carbohydrates.

Training Foods

In training, however, when the athlete may be concentrating on increased muscle and mass size, protein requirements are increased. The high school athlete, who is competing and growing at the same time, needs more protein than an adult. Certain foods must be included in the daily diet: large portions of meat, cheese, fish, or eggs; three or more glasses of milk; a variety of vegetables, particularly yellow and green; fruits and citrus; and generous amounts of enriched, whole-grain breads and cereals. Milk is a good source of top-quality protein, calcium, phosphorus, and riboflavin. To break up the monotony of beef as a source of protein, various cuts of lamb, pork, or chicken may be substituted.

As in the case of regular eating habits a diversity of foods should be incorporated. From the standpoint of morale it is often necessary to include a "forbidden" food such as pie à la mode on special occasions. A rigid diet sometimes has a more deleterious effect than "cheating" on occasion. As long as the diet is normally well balanced, it is all right occasionally to include cakes, pies, gravies, and other foods that ordinarily must not be eaten.

It is generally not advisable to eat just before or just after physical exertion. The primary reason for this is that the energy normally necessary for the activity is diverted to be used for digestion, absorption, and utilization of the food. And exercise diverts the blood from digestion processes. Thus, the energy output is divided, decreasing the efficiency of both physical activity and digestion.

It is also important that great amounts of fluids not be consumed just prior to or following periods of strenuous activity. And when they are taken, they should be moderate in temperature—neither too hot nor too cold. When liquids are taken in extreme temperatures, the system is thrown into slight shock, thereby diverting the remainder of the body from its normal efficiency range.

Eating Schedules

Several practical eating schedules might be suggested for any sport. For example, when contests or activities are held in the evening, the major meal should be taken in the morning. In the morning the digestive system and nutritional state of the body are at a low ebb. A substantial amount of food energy is needed to carry out the day's normal activities. This gap between the large morning meal and the evening athletics leaves enough time for the proper digestion, absorption, and utilization of food.

A good breakfast should include generous portions of protein food, which may be bacon, beef patties, ham and eggs, along with fruit or fruit juice, whole-grain toast, and milk. The noon meal may be composed of more easily digested protein foods, such as eggs, milk, lean meat, and fish. Under ideal conditions exercise should not be engaged in until three or four hours have elapsed since the ingestion of this meal. Then the digestive tract will be totally free of food, and the entire reserve of the body can be used for athletic activity.

If the strenuous activity is in the afternoon, say at 2 P.M., only one meal, at 9 or 10 A.M., should be eaten. This meal should consist of easily digested, satisfying foods: fruit or fruit juice, soft-boiled eggs, broiled meat (fried or greasy foods increase digestion time), cottage cheese, whole-grain bread, and butter. Of course, overeating should be avoided at all times.

An hour or two after the game or event another meal can be consumed, depending on whether or not the digestive tract is out of its nervous condition brought on by the activity. This meal should be good-sized and well balanced, including fruit, meat, vegetables, salad, and whole-grain bread.

FOOD GROUPS

The guarantee of a balanced diet is foods taken from each group every day. The following is a list of the food groups and their components:

Meat group
(Each sample contains approximately 8 grams of protein, 75 calories, and 6 grams of fat)

> 5 oz. steak
> ¼ cup tuna, lobster, or salmon
> 5 small oysters or clams
> 1 slice of cheese (¼" thick)
> ¼ cup cottage cheese
> 4 medium sardines
> 1 egg

Deep-yellow or dark-green vegetables (half-cup servings)

Broccoli	Beet greens
Chicory	Chard
Carrots	Collards
Pumpkins	Dandelions

Peppers
Tomatoes
Winter squash
Watercress

Kale
Mustard greens
Spinach
Turnip greens
Lettuce

Fruits
Apples
Apricots
Bananas
Blueberries
Cherries
Dates
Figs
Grapes
Honeydew melons

Papayas
Peaches
Pears
Pineapples
Plums
Raisins
Prunes
Watermelon
Mangos

Citrus fruits
Oranges
Grapefruit
Cantaloupe

Strawberries
Tangerines
Tomato juice

Vegetables (half-cup servings)
Asparagus
Beets
Brussels sprouts
Cabbage
Cauliflower
Celery
Cucumbers
Eggplant
Mushrooms

Okra
Onions
Green peas
Radishes
Rutabagas
Sauerkraut
Stringbeans
Summer squash
Turnips

Fats (One tablespoon contains 5 grams of fat and 45 calories)

Bacon
Butter or margarine

Cream
Cream cheese
Dressing
Mayonnaise
Oil or cooking fat

Milk

(1 cup of whole milk contains 12 grams of carbohydrate, 8 grams of protein, 10 grams of fat, and 170 calories)

The milk group of foods should be included generously in all diets. Milk provides the essential calcium for teeth and bone growth, protein for tissue repair and growth, along with essential minerals. Milk is high in riboflavin, which keeps skin healthy and clear.

Considering all that milk has to offer, it is relatively low in calories. One cup (8 ounces) of milk contains about 110 calories, one cup of skim milk about 90 calories.

The Consumer and Food Economics Research Department of the U.S. Government recommends the daily amounts of milk as in Table 3.2.

These quantities vary according to the individual or from whom information of this sort is gathered. It happens that this is a rather functional chart that we agree with.

Table 3.3 lists the approximate number of calories contained in one cup (8 ounces) of selected milk and other dairy

TABLE 3.2
RECOMMENDED DAILY ALLOWANCES OF MILK

AGE GROUP	8-OZ. CUPS
children under 9	2 or 3
children, 9–12	3 or more
teenagers	4 or more
adults	2 or more
pregnant women over 19	3 or more
nursing mothers over 19	4 or more

products.Table 3.4 gives the approximate number of calories in one tablespoon of milk products.

Cheese also supplies the important mineral calcium. A slice of cheese (1 ounce), cheddar type, is equivalent to ¾ cup of whole milk; 1 cup of cottage cheese equals 1/3 cup of whole milk; 2 tablespoons of cream cheese equals 1 tablespoon of whole milk. In normal cases we advise the use of whole milk. Nature has provided the necessary amounts of magnesium and fat needed to assimilate the calcium in milk. If this natural proportion is altered, as in the case of low-fat or skimmed milk, the tendency for calcium to be poorly absorbed is increased. Hypercalcification, or calcium buildup, causes the formation of painful calcium deposits in the ureter and kidneys. Unless obesity demands the intake of low-fat dairy products, whole milk should be used.

Supplements and Necessities

Iron-rich foods such as liver, prunes, oysters, raisins, apricots, and dried beans and peas should be used often in the diet. We also suggest supplementing these with desiccated liver tablets and yeast tablets, which will provide that extra spark of the vital B vitamins to the diet. In these times of processed, denatured foods a dietary increase such as these supplements is a cheap and effective way of maximizing the dietary regime.

GOOD DIETARY HABITS

In order for this information to have any relevance, athletes must take into consideration their dietary habits.

It is helpful for all people, but again especially athletes, to periodically check their food intake and diet. It would be impossible to watch yourself constantly, but every month or so it is a good idea to check your diet for two or three days. Naturally, honesty is of prime importance. You must stick to your usual diet, and just list all the foods you eat for three

TABLE 3.3
CALORIES IN 8 OUNCES OF DAIRY PRODUCTS

MILK

Buttermilk, made from skim milk	90
Chocolate milk, made from whole milk and chocolate	210
Chocolate-flavored drink, made from lowfat milk and cocoa	190
Dry (mixed with water):	
Nonfat	90
Whole	160
Evaporated (diluted with equal volume of water):	
Skim	90
Whole	170
Fresh skim or lowfat:	
Lowfat (1 percent milkfat)	110
Skim (nonfat)	90
2 percent	130
2 percent (added nonfat milk solids)	145
Fresh whole, homogenized	160
Sweetened condensed, undiluted	980
Yogurt, made from partially skimmed milk	125

HALF-AND-HALF

Half-and-half (11 percent milkfat)	325
Sour half-and-half (11 percent milkfat)	325

CREAM

Sour (18 percent milkfat)	485
Table or coffee (18 percent milkfat)	505
Whipping (unwhipped):	
Heavy (36 percent milkfat)	840
Light (30 percent milkfat)	715

FROZEN DESSERTS

Frozen custard (10 percent milkfat)	255
Ice cream, plain (10 percent milkfat)	255
Ice cream, rich (16 percent milkfat)	330
Ice milk (5 percent milkfat)	200
Ice milk, soft-serve (5 percent milkfat)	265
Sherbet, fruit (1.2 percent milkfat)	260

*The number of calories in frozen desserts varies with the amount of milkfat in the mix and the volume of air incorporated into the product during processing.

TABLE 3.4
CALORIES IN 1 TABLESPOON OF DAIRY PRODUCTS

MILK		
Dry:		
Nonfat, instant (dry)	15	
Whole, instant (dry)	20	
Evaporated (whole, undiluted)	20	
Fresh skim	5	
Fresh whole, homogenized	10	
Sweetened condensed (undiluted)	60	
Yogurt, made from partially skimmed milk	10	
HALF-AND-HALF		
Half-and-half (11 percent milkfat)	20	
Sour half-and-half (11 percent milkfat)	20	
CREAM		
Sour (18 percent milkfat)	30	
Table or coffee (18 percent milkfat)	30	
Whipping (unwhipped):		
Heavy (36 percent milkfat)	55	
Light (30 percent milkfat)	45	

days. Then, only at the end of the experiment, tabulate the results (use the chart at the end of this book to calculate the calories, fats, and carbohydrates).

If you are unhappy with the tabulations, make the appropriate adjustments and try to stick to them with the aid of a chart such as the sample in Table 3.5.

Because snacks are an essential part of the American diet, it is imperative for athletes to choose snacks with full nutritional value. Unfortunately, it seems that Americans are preoccupied with junk foods—those with high sugar and low nutrient content.

Everyone has occasionally eaten foods that are high in sugar, loaded calories, or with little nutritional value. It has been demonstrated that excess sugar leads to problems in the nervous system, digestive disorders, and problems related to vitamin B-complex deficiencies. Sugar can satisfy hunger, too, thus preventing the body from getting full-value nutrients. We are not advocating the elimination of natural carbohydrates or sugars such as those found in fruits, but the average American gets too much refined sugar. Junk foods are high

TABLE 3.5

A RECORD OF DAILY FOOD INTAKE

	FOOD	CALORIES	PROTEIN	FAT	CARB.
Breakfast					
Morning snack					
Lunch					
Afternoon snack					
Dinner					
Evening snack					
Extras					
Total					

TABLE 3.6
SUGAR CONTENT OF COMMON SNACK FOODS

FOOD	SERVING	SUGAR EQUIVALENT (IN TEASPOONS)
Cake		
Angel	1 piece	6
Chocolate	2 layer with icing	15
iced cream puff	1 custard-filled	5
plain doughnut	3 inches in diameter	4
Candy		
chocolate fudge	1½ inch square	4
chocolate bar	small bar	7
Lifesavers	one	½
Cookies		
brownies	2 inch square	3
macaroons	one large	3
Ice cream		
regular vanilla	⅛ quart	6
Pie		
apple	1/6 of a medium pie	12
cherry	same	14
coconut custard	same	10
pumpkin	same	10
Soft drinks		
Coca-Cola	one 6-ounce bottle	4½
Ginger ale	same	4½

in sugar and low in vitamins and minerals that aid in the absorption of nutrients. Table 3.6 lists a number of common foods with their approximate sugar content in teaspoons.

Dr. Carlton Fredericks claims that a high-carbohydrate diet lengthens convalescence in respiratory infections and predisposes a person to common colds and sinus problems. The more desirable carbohydrates are those that also supply vitamins, minerals, and protein—foods such as whole-grain cereals, bread, and brown rice. Table 3.7 shows the imbalance of calories to protein value in a sampling of some common snack foods.

Although it is practically impossible to eliminate all junk

TABLE 3.7

CALORIES AND PROTEIN VALUE OF COMMON SNACK FOODS

	SIZE OF PORTION	CALORIES	PROTEIN (GRAMS)
Candy bar, milk chocolate	1 small bar (⅞ ounce)	130	2
Fondant mints or patties	1 average (40 to pound)	40	—
Chocolate creams	1 average (35 to pound)	50	—
Fudge, plain	1 piece, 1" square	100	—
Peanut brittle	1 piece, 2½ × 2½ × ⅜"	110	2
Gumdrops	1 large or 8 small	35	—
Marshmallows	1 average (60 to pound)	25	—
Cookies, plain	2 small or 1 large	120	1
Cookies, oatmeal	2 small or 1 large	115	2
Wafers, as vanilla	2 small, thin	30	—
Cupcake, not iced	1 medium, 2¾" diameter	145	2
Cupcake, iced	1 medium, 2¾" diameter	185	2
Brownies	1 piece, 2 × 2 × ¾"	140	2
Cake, not iced	Med. piece, 2 × 3 × 1½"	200	4
Cake, chocolate icing	Med. piece, 1/16 10" cake	370	3
Cake, angel food or sponge	Small piece, 2" sector	115	1
Doughnut	1 medium	125	1
Eclair, chocolate	1 average	315	8
Pie, fruit	1/7 medium-size pie	350	3
Pie, custard type	1/7 medium-size pie	280	8
Pudding, cornstarch, vanilla	½ cup	140	5
Pudding, rice with raisins	½ cup	160	5
Fruit betty	½ cup	175	2
Prune whip	½ cup	100	2
Custard	½ cup	145	7
Gelatin dessert with fruit	½ cup	80	2
Milkshake, chocolate	Fountain size (5 oz. milk, 2 small scoops ice cream, 2 tablespoons sirup)	340	8
Cocoa, all milk	1 table-size cup (6 oz. milk)	175	7
Sundaes	1 medium, 2 tbsp. topping	240	3
Sodas	Fountain size	260	2
Carbonated drinks	1 large glass (8 oz.)	95	—
Lemonade, lightly sweetened	1 large glass (10 oz.)	130	—
Ginger ale	1 large glass (8 oz.)	70	—

foods, it is not difficult to understand their disadvantages and therefore to make a conscious effort to avoid them. They do little for the athlete except to add extra weight and create physiological disturbances. Young athletes, especially, have the chance to develop long-time healthy nutritional habits and avoid the American "sugarholic" syndrome.

4 TRAINING AND NUTRITION

Part of the athlete's life-style is training, and one of the greatest concerns of the athlete is weight control. In some sports weight increase is desirable; in others weight loss is key. Many people think training is only for competing athletes —a preparation for a particular event or game, but in reality all people should be in training, exercising to keep physically fit.

WHAT TRAINING CAN DO

At one time a person who was free of disease was considered physically fit. This definition does not hold true any longer. To be physically fit in contemporary terms one must have full use of lungs, a sound cardiovascular system, and good muscle tone. These are all necessary to maintain maximum interaction with nature and society. The process that strives to achieve the greatest use of the body and the physical potential is called *training*.

It does not matter what this training is intended for, whether it be the preparation of a child for adulthood, the development of a handicapped individual, routine exercise for the middle-aged or the elderly, or preparation for athletic competition on an amateur or professional level. These all require the essential aims and methods of training.

Numerous physiological responses can be changed by

training. It has been estimated that a regular training program can lead to approximately a 25-percent improvement in the individual bodily system and up to a 100-percent improvement in the magnitude and duration of the work that can be done. It has been demonstrated that persons who exercise or train regularly resist fatigue better and are capable of greater efforts than their sedentary counterparts.

Improvements from Training

Eight major changes are brought about by training:

1. Increased mechanical efficiency (that is, lower oxygen consumption for a given amount of work).

2. Greater muscular strength and improved neuromuscular coordination.

3. A higher maximum cardiac output with less of an increase in pulse rate and blood pressure during exercise.

4. Increased oxygen consumption.

5. Lower blood lactate for a given amount of energy output.

6. Increased maximum pulmonary ventilation.

7. Improved heat dissipation during energy expenditure.

8. Quicker recovery in pulse rate and blood pressure after prolonged energy output.

The degree to which these alterations occur will determine the improvement in the individual's general fitness.

Restrictions

The amount of training one does, of course, depends on the amount of energy one must expend. The person who leads

a rather sedentary life certainly does not need the same training program as does a pro football player. On the other hand,
increased training may bring to the inactive individual an
increased feeling of well-being and improved health of body
and mind.

The size of an individual's heart, which influences to a
great degree the maximum energy output, varies according
to the size and amount of the individual's skeletal muscle.
Normally, then, a very muscular person has a very muscular
heart; a great deal of energy output is expected of this individual. The variation of this rule occurs if the heart has some sort
of pulmonary lesion that restricts physical exertion to whatever the fault or condition may accommodate.

The first prerequisite of training is to make certain by
physical examination and by study of the individual's medical
history that there are no pathological lesions of the vascular,
pulmonary, or excretory systems that would interfere with
and restrict muscular activity. If lesions do occur and alterations are not made accordingly, training can be carried so far
as to increase damage to the individual.

Strength, Endurance, Speed, and Skill

Various muscles and muscle groupings develop and de-
generate disproportionately to each other. It has been
noted that a strength factor registers in children around 4
or 5 years of age. A younger child cannot realize the fruits
of directed effort. Nature has devised a time system
whereby, under ordinary circumstances, the muscles
needed to maintain an upright position and the muscles
needed for mastication develop faster and better in relation
to the others. These include the calf and back muscles and
the front surface of the hip and neck. At about 13 or 14
the strength level almost reaches the adult equivalent, and
in some cases this figure exceeds it. Generally, maximum
strength occurs between 20 and 25.

This disproportion is true of decreasing strength as well.
For example, the muscles of the stomach, back surface of the

hip, and the extensors of the arm grow old and lose their strength earliest of all.

Endurance factors are generally related to age. Endurance is extremely good at around 9 to 13, after which any further development depends on physical training, physical makeup, and psychological motivation.

Reaction time is also related to age. This development occurs first in the fingers, feet, and neck, and later in hip and body movement. The highest level of speed reaction can be reached at about 18 to 20 yrs. After 25 or 30, and until 50 or 60, the function of speed and strength of various muscle groups only gradually worsens. (This is especially true in the case of abdominal muscles.) But sometime during the fifties or sixties there is a sharp deterioration in neuromuscular activity. All of this is naturally dependent on how much exercise each muscle group gets.

The task of training is to obtain harmonious development and conservation of strength, speed, and endurance of various groups of muscles. This involves the correct application of physical and dietary patterns according to the individual's particular needs and by the presence of any pathological conditions, whether acquired or congenital.

Strength, speed, endurance, and skill are needed for any effective athletic endeavor. It is during the training period that athletes must develop these qualities, either collectively or with stress on one or another. For example, strength would be stressed over the others in training for power events such as shot put or weight lifting; in events such as sprinting speed is required over strength; in long-distance running greater development of endurance is needed.

This may be an oversimplification, because all sports overlap to some degree and require a rather ill-defined amount of all these qualities.

The development of strength depends on exercise against great resistance, as in weight lifting; speed is developed by exercising for short periods at maximum rate; endurance is developed by exercising against comparatively low resistance for a long time; skill is acquired when a constantly repeated pattern becomes a conditioned reflex. Training demands all these types of exercise. If there are specific needs, the training program should highlight exercises that develop these areas.

Training can be an end in itself, for its inherent physical and psychological value. On the other hand, if one is involved in athletics on a competitive level, then training is simply a means to an end. Training alone does not ensure victory. An individual who competes must give his all in the game as well as in training.

Training is a never-ending process. It is the nourishment of fitness; without training, fitness dies.

No matter what demands are made on the physical, there is always the psychological motivation to be considered. This aspect of training is of paramount importance. It is always easier to accomplish something when you want to and when you believe you can.

As the training develops the physical virtues, it stimulates the psychological ones. As individuals experience an increased sense of well-being and see the marked physical changes, they get a feeling of self-improvement that in turn promotes greater interest in training. These changes are always more apparent in the early stages. As training develops, they will not be quite so marked. It is thus possible for *anyone*, within the bounds of his or her particular physiology, to attain a high standard of performance in a relatively short time.

The time to train for competition is not just prior to the event. Preseason conditioning programs should start long before preseason practice. The coaching staff must see that every athlete is primed well in advance, for optimum performance and efficiency.

The Results of Training
Training produces various effects on the different systems of the body. The effect on the muscles includes an in-

crease in size of the skeletal muscles. Authorities seem to agree that muscle fiber is not formed by exercise, but is simply developed to full size by it. This size increase is accompanied by an increase in the number of capillaries in the muscle. In strength exercises such as weight lifting the muscle fiber develops to an excessive degree (hypertrophy), whereas in exercises for endurance such as long-distance running the number of capillaries in the muscles is increased. This increase allows a greater amount of oxygen and nutrients to enter the organs, thus maintaining the maximum functioning ability of that tissue. As a result of all this there is an increase in strength in several areas: (1) the capacity to create more powerful muscular contractions, therefore a gain in power; (2) the ability to repeat contractions more rapidly, therefore an increase in speed; (3) the ability to maintain for a longer stretch of time, which is an increase in endurance. The strength of the muscles can be increased only by exercising them against increasing resistance to weight and/or moving the body at higher speeds. During early training it is possible to increase muscle strength by three or more times without a proportional volume increase.

The end result of training on the muscle depends on the kind of exercise performed, speed, duration, degree of repetition, and intensity of contractions. Individual bodily characteristics also determine the development of muscle tissue, so that no two persons utilizing the same training regime will develop similarly. An increase in muscular strength does not bring about an increase in endurance. Comparing a muscular weight lifter and a mile runner, the former has an obvious strength advantage, but the endurance of the runner exceeds that of the weight lifter.

Training also improves the transmission of nerve impulses to the muscle fiber. This results in a greater number of fibers responding, thereby causing maximum strength. Thus, it appears that training increases muscular efficiency both chemically and electrically.

The effect of training on the respiratory system reaches

its peak after progressive training of from four to six weeks. Because of improved neuromuscular functioning, oxygen consumption and carbon dioxide production decrease progressively as the training proceeds. As exercise causes the pulmonary ventilation to be reduced, the labor required for breathing decreases and the amount of blood needed to maintain those muscles decreases. Naturally, the muscles of respiration, not only the diaphragm but also the thoracic and abdominal muscles, become stronger and more efficient during training. As is true of all the effects of training, their improvement is proportional to the duration and quality of the exercise performed.

Training and Neuromuscular Coordination

The precision and economy of any action involved in athletic activity is improved by training. It also eliminates any unnecessary static or dynamic muscular contraction, and eventually the responses of the body become more reflexive and less voluntary. As a result, for any given performance a decrease in energy output occurs that can conceivably reach one-quarter of the total energy necessary for the action before training. For any athletic performance there is a specific motion that is the most efficient and that requires the least oxygen consumption. Training results in the harnessing of this specific motion to the activity requiring it.

It should be obvious that proper nervous system reactions are needed for the body to make the necessary internal adjustments to exercise. Fundamentally, all systems of the body in some way or other rely on the efficient functioning of the nervous system. In fact, the entire relationship of the body to its environment depends on the nervous system. Activity or movement of any sort is the product of muscular coordination brought about by impulses from the nervous system. The greater the degree of coordination needed for a specific movement, the greater is the precision of the movement.

Many of our daily activities are carried out subconsciously. When a person walks, the pace, duration, stops, and starts are all under the control of conscious desire, but the actual process of placing one foot in front of the other is an unconscious, automatic response referred to as a conditioned reflex. These patterns are learned by the central nervous system (CNS) and remain established for periods long surviving their use. This is the reason that one never forgets how to swim or how to ride a bike. They are the result of conditioned reflexes.

If one were to stop and think about which movements are most economical for catching a ball, for example, the action would be hampered by the relatively slow-acting intellectual center. When the body responds to conditioned reflex, however, no thought takes place. The body reacts automatically, and the action occurs smoothly and efficiently. These patterns that develop as a result of training are dependent on the nervous system.

For optimal performance these reflexes must be so highly developed that they do not break down under stress or fatigue. Once established, they remain a pattern though their functioning ability may vary from day to day. This variation occurs not as a result of a lack of skill, but rather from a lack of total integration of conditioned reflexes. When this occurs, it is often referred to as an "off day" by athletes. It all depends on a complex network of circumstances originating in both the psychological and physiological components of motivation.

The development of skill depends on the formation of functional circuits in the CNS. It stands to reason that the more complex the skill, the more complex is the necessary circuitry, and so more of training is required in order to perform complex functions efficiently. This is generally achieved by repetition of the movement, which wears a path in the electrical circuits of the CNS. It is important that pattern formation begin slowly, to facilitate the correction of any deviations or mistakes. It is always more difficult to break a bad habit than to create a new one. After a time the body will learn to accommodate this new action; it will become second nature, so to speak.

Training and the Cardiovascular System

The heart becomes more efficient when it can circulate more blood while beating less frequently. As the training progresses, the heart becomes stronger, emptying itself more thoroughly during each contraction, which impels blood outward (systole). Cardiac output and stroke volume are also increased. It is not exceptional for the resting pulse rate to be reduced by 10 to 20 beats per minute between the beginning and end of a training period. Increased heart efficiency and strength bring a proportionately greater amount of oxygen and fuel to the system, thus allowing individuals to reach higher levels of performance.

Another aspect of the cardiovascular system affected by training is blood pressure. Initially in the untrained individual there is a progressive fall of the systolic pressure, which precedes exhaustion. This effect is gradually retarded by training, because the individual becomes more capable of doing increased work for longer periods without appreciable variation in the blood pressure. There is also a change in the recovery period after exercise. The more trained the individual, the quicker his heart rate and pressure return to the pre-exercise level.

The amount of oxygen needed by the working muscles is reduced as a result of training, and in turn the necessary blood flow to these muscles is decreased. Thus, "extra" blood is available for the functioning efficiency of other organs. This equilibrium in blood distribution is crucially important when exercising in warm or hot surroundings. When more blood is available, heat dissipation in the skin is more effective, and the body temperature remains lower because evaporation is a cooling process.

Table 4.1 shows differences in cardiac output between the trained and the untrained.

The final aspect of improved cardiovascular response to

TABLE 4.1
CARDIAC OUTPUT DIFFERENCES BETWEEN TRAINED
AND UNTRAINED SUBJECTS

	Stroke at Rest	Volume at Work	Pulse Rate at Work
UNTRAINED	60ml	120ml	180 per minute
TRAINED	100ml	200ml	107 per minute

training is the increased efficiency and strength of the intra-abdominal and intra-thoracic pressure. The heart's pumping effect is assisted by this pressure, and so the large job of blood distribution is eased, thereby saving wear and tear on the heart.

Rates of Improvement

Soon after regular training begins, the respiratory rate, the heart rate, and the blood lactic acid all decrease. After an organized exercise routine has been followed for a few weeks, no further improvement occurs. In order for additional improvements to occur the *duration* of the daily training must be increased because the work rate remains the same. In other words, if one runs one mile a day for two weeks, a general improvement of bodily functions occurs and then levels off. However, if after this leveling point the same time is spent running without an increase in distance, the improvements will not continue. If the work rate (speed) remains the same but the distance (duration) is increased, improvement will continue. This improvement is expressed in lower heart and respiratory rates and by a reduction in blood lactic acid. The periodic addition of this type of scheme to the training regime will guarantee improvement until a point is reached that can be called a state of maximum training. This of course varies from individual to individual, according to the dictates of the body and mind.

Tests have shown that when a moderate level of training

is interrupted for a period of time from a week to ten days, there is no evidence of any regression. On the other hand, if *heavy* training is interrupted for from four to six days, there is a subsequent increase of lactic acid in the blood and a faster heart rate occurs, all adding up to a decrease in efficiency. The individual who trains just to keep active should maintain a moderate amount of exercise. This is especially true of the middle-aged or older person, whose chances of cardiac problems are more pronounced. In the case of professional or serious amateur competitors, of course, heavy training schedules are virtually mandatory.

Specific training prepares an untrained person for specific athletic functioning. A power lifter will use weights during training, while a distance runner will use track event training. This is not to say that one will not do the other, but simply that one stresses one activity over the other. It has been observed that when people, regardless of the quality and condition of their bodies, perform exercises for which they are not specifically trained, maximum lactic acid saturation is reached more readily and exhaustion and fatigue appear sooner. This suggests that the training process occurs partly in the muscles themselves.

Training Plans

In making a plan for training, it is important to consider such characteristics as relative capacities, sex, and age. It is absurd for females to train unilaterally with males for power-lifting events, or for a 250-pound male to compete with a female of diminutive stature in the sprint. Age and physical shape are rather obvious restrictions, though it has been shown that *any* healthy individuals can modify their physiological efficiency with training—up to a point. Even strenuous training under ideal conditions will enable an athlete to reach and maintain a maximum that is relative to the capabilities of the individual. We all can't be Larry Csonkas or Billie Jean Kings even though we may train just as strenuously as they. Overtraining often leads to staleness and chronic fatigue, a point of diminishing returns characterized by greater concen-

TABLE 4.2
IDEAL WEIGHTS FOR WOMEN

Height (with shoes on) 2-inch heels Feet	Inches	Small frame	Medium frame	Large frame
4	10	92–98	96–107	104–119
4	11	94–101	98–110	106–122
5	0	96–104	101–113	109–125
5	1	99–107	104–116	112–128
5	2	102–110	107–119	115–131
5	3	105–113	110–122	118–134
5	4	108–116	113–126	121–138
5	5	111–119	116–130	125–142
5	6	114–123	120–135	129–146
5	7	118–127	124–139	133–150
5	8	122–131	128–143	137–154
5	9	126–135	132–147	141–158
5	10	130–140	136–151	145–163
5	11	134–144	140–155	149–168
6	0	138–148	144–159	153–173

Note: Age 25 and over. For those between 18 and 25, deduct one pound for each year under 25. Weights include indoor clothing.

TABLE 4.3
IDEAL WEIGHTS FOR MEN

Height (with shoes on) 1-inch heels Feet	Inches	Small frame	Medium frame	Large frame
5	2	112–120	118–129	126–141
5	3	115–123	121–133	129–144
5	4	118–126	124–136	132–148
5	5	121–129	127–139	135–152
5	6	124–133	130–143	138–156
5	7	128–137	134–147	142–161
5	8	132–141	138–152	147–166
5	9	136–145	142–156	151–170
5	10	140–150	146–160	155–174
5	11	144–154	150–165	159–179
6	0	148–158	154–170	164–184
6	1	152–162	158–175	168–189
6	2	156–167	162–180	173–194
6	3	160–171	167–185	178–199
6	4	164–175	172–190	182–204

Note: Age 25 and over. Weights include indoor clothing.

trations of lactic acid and a higher heart rate than previously noted during the training program.

Although everyone can improve their own working capacity, outstanding athletic performance is attainable by only a few. These individuals have highly efficient and precisely integrated physiological mechanisms. They are born with mental and physical capabilities that can be developed through precise and effective training to make possible superior athletic performances. It is said that nature makes no mistakes. Each of us must take an honest account of what we have and develop athletic activities within that framework. When conscientious application of controlled individualized training is made, the results will be highly rewarding for all.

WEIGHT CONTROL

In order to derive maximum benefits from training it is important to achieve proper weight. The ideal is within one or two pounds of the prescribed weights in Tables 4.2 and 4.3.

The Problem of Obesity

Obesity is common among all age groups in the United States. Its most tragic aspect is the attendant risk of heart failure and other weight-related medical problems. An article in the *Maine Medical Association Journal* (May 1973) states that in our highly technological society the risk of infectious diseases that was high 25 years ago is now rather low. However, other ailments now pose a greater threat, especially heart disease, cardiovascular diseases, and cancer.

Of particular importance is the relationship of obesity to increased mortality and lowered life expectancy. This is especially true of the members of this group in the 40–50 age bracket. Obesity is directly associated with hypertension and myocardial failure which accounts for a majority of the tragic deaths of men at the apex of their success. In fact, a long-term study of some 5,000 people showed that obese persons develop cardiovascular diseases about 80% more frequently than person of normal weight and diabetes about 70% more frequently. After age 45, person who are 10 lbs. overweight are subject to an 8% increase in death rate; 20 lbs., 18%; 30 lbs., 28%; 50 lbs., 56%. The importance of these statistics is to emphasize the deleterious effects of obesity. More important than statistics is that the majority of cases of obesity are potentially preventable.

The article claims that "half of the population or more than 100 million Americans are too fat!"

Some of the reasons for overweight are abnormal functions of the thyroid, hypothalamus, pituitary, adrenal, and sex glands. But these physiological factors cause only a small percentage of all obesity. The major reason is lack of exercise and eating too much.

The article continues, enumerating the devastating effects of obesity.

An increase in vascular circulation resulting in an increased demand on the heart. In addition, there is the constant association of elevated blood pressure commonly called hypertension. Fat is also infiltrated into cardiac muscle, putting further demand on the cardiovascular system. In the same fashion, there are fatty deposits in the walls of the blood vessels, a condition called atherosclerosis. This predisposes to myocardial infarcts or "heart attacks" and cerebrovascular accidents or "strokes." The increased weight in itself results in degenerative arthritis of the joints. There is also increased infection in the skin beneath the fat. Thrombophlebitis and varicose veins are also commonly associated factors.

How to Lose Weight

To combat this problem of obesity the American Heart Association has five suggestions, published in their bulletin "Diet and Coronary Heart Disease."

1. A caloric intake adjusted to achieve and maintain ideal body weight.

2. A reduction in total fat calories achieved by a substantial reduction in dietary saturated fatty acids. Reduction from the usual 40–45 percent of total calories obtained from fat to no more than 35 percent is desirable.

3. A substantial reduction in dietary cholesterol to an average daily intake of approximately 300 milligrams.

4. An increase in foods containing complex natural carbohydrates, such as vegetables, fruits, cereals, and a decrease in use of refined sugar, including that contained in candy, soft drinks, and other sweets.

5. The avoidance of excessive salt intake.

Obesity is always detrimental to the physiological well-being of athletes. Weight loss must be incorporated with basic common sense attitudes, underscored by solid information. Exercise must be employed daily throughout one's life. We must start young by pursuing sports that can be enjoyed through most of life. Among such sports are golf, swimming, tennis, handball, cross-country, volleyball, skiing, bicycling, and jogging.

If you feel that you're too heavy, the best way to lose weight is slowly—and begin now! According to the AMA Americans' pursuit of instant weight reduction has made them prey to every gimmick on the market. Essentially, the only reliable way to lose weight is a regular training program and a reduced intake of calories and carbohydrates.

The body is an efficient organism that remorselessly changes excess calories into accumulations of fat. As we stated earlier, one pound of fat is equal to about 3,500 extra calories. There just isn't any way around the fact that calories in excess of what the body needs for energy expenditure will invariably be turned into fat.

Low-carbohydrate diets seem to work, probably because high-calorie foods are usually high-carbohydrate foods, too—for example, one piece of chocolate cake has 445 calories and 70 grams of carbohydrate. This exceeds the recommended daily allotment of a low-carbohydrate diet by 20 grams.

If one rations the intake of carbohydrates and calories conscientiously, weight loss will soon follow. Beyond this, it appears that when carbohydrates and calories are restricted, the salt and water carried by the body are decreased, thereby creating an even faster rate of weight loss. The United States Air Force Academy has designed a diet that keeps carbohydrate intake to between 40 and 50 grams per day. This means that weight loss for a large person can be aided by not exceeding a daily intake of about 50 grams and for smaller persons about 40 grams. Ideally the daily allotment of carbohydrates should be ingested from "wholesome" foods like dairy products, vegetables and fruit, rather than "empty" carbohydrates such as pastry and candies.

Table 4.4 contains a list of food choices, their carbohydrate content in grams. Many good foods such as meat, vegetables, and cheese are acceptable on this diet, therefore ensuring satisfying, tasty meals.

The Air Force Academy recommends running exercises in association with this diet—this seems appropriate because it requires little skill and therefore can be performed by everyone. It must be remembered that pace length, leg length, and speed are not important for weight loss. What is important is daily observance of energy expenditure. In this case if a daily caloric expenditure of 100 calories is maintained, there will be approximately 10 pounds of weight loss in one year.

TABLE 4.4
CARBOHYDRATE CONTENT OF COMMON FOODS

FOOD	HOUSEHOLD MEASURE	GRAMS
Milk		
whole milk	8 ounces	11.8
ice cream	half-pint	14.8
Cheese		
American cheese	1 ounce	0.5
cottage cheese	1 rounded tablespoon	1.3
Fats		
bacon	3 strips	0.0
butter	1 tablespoon	0.0
french dressing	1 tablespoon	1.9
margarine	—	0.0
salad oil	—	0.0
mayonnaise	1 tablespoon	0.2
Eggs		
1 egg	—	0.73
Meat		
bologna	2 slices	1.00
frankfurter	1	1.9
hash	1 serving	7.0
chicken, turkey, ham, veal, beef, lamb, pork	1 serving	0.0
Nuts		
Mixed	10/15	3.0
Fish		
Oysters	4/6	1.2
Shrimp	5/6	0.5
Vegetables (fresh)		
Asparagus	6 stalks	2.0
Beans, green	½ cup	2.0
Beans, lima	½ cup	23.5
Beet greens	½ cup	5.6
Beets	2 medium	9.7
Broccoli	½ cup	5.6
Brussels sprouts	6	6.2
Cabbage	⅔ cup, cooked	5.3
Carrots	1 large	9.3
Cauliflower	4 tablespoons	3.4
Celery	2 stalks	1.9

TABLE 4.4 (con't)

FOOD	HOUSEHOLD MEASURE	GRAMS
Corn	1 ear	20.0
Cucumber	½	¼
Eggplant	½ cup, cooked	5.6
Kale	½ cup, cooked	7.2
Lettuce	5 leaves	0.9
Lettuce	¼ head	1.8
Okra	6 pods	19.0
Onions	⅔ small	10.3
Green peas	½ cup	17.7
Green peppers	1	5.7
Potatoes	1 small	19.1
Spinach	½ cup, cooked	3.2
Squash	½ cup	7.1
Tomatoes	1 medium	0.4
Turnips	½ cup	7.1
Catsup	1 tablespoon	4.8
Tomato juice	1 cup	4.3
Fruit		
Apples	1 large	22.4
Apricots	2–3	12.9
Avocado	½	5.1
Banana	1 small	23.0
Strawberries	10 large	8.1
Other berries	⅔ cup	15.1
Cantaloupe	½ melon	6.9
Grapefruit	½ small	10.1
Grapes	22	16.7
Lemons	1 medium	8.7
Orange	1 small	11.2
Orange juice	½ cup	12.9
Peach	1 medium	12.0
Pear	1 medium	15.8
Pineapple	½ cup	13.7
Plums	3 medium	12.9
Rhubarb	1 cup	3.8
Watermelon	1 slice (6″ × 1½″)	41.4
Canned Fruit		
Cherries	½ cup	20.0

TABLE 4.4 (con't)

FOOD	HOUSEHOLD MEASURE	GRAMS
Cranberry sauce	1 tablespoon	10.2
Pineapple in syrup	1 slice	21.1
Dried Fruit		
Apricots	4–6	20.0
Prunes	2–3	21.3
Flour Meal		
Corn meal	½ cup	15.7
Cornstarch	1 tablespoon	10.0
Cereals		
Cornflakes	1 cup	18.0
Oatmeal	½ cup, cooked	13.0
Puffed Rice	¾ cup	8.6
Shredded wheat	1 biscuit	24.0
Spaghetti, macaroni	½ cup	14.8
Noodles	½ cup	14.8
White rice	½ cup, cooked	15.8
Tapioca	1 tablespoon	12.9
Sugars		
Honey	1 tablespoon	15.0
Jam	1 level tablespoon	14.2
Jellies	1 level tablespoon	13.0
Brown sugar	1 tablespoon	10.5
Granulated sugar	1 tablespoon	5.0
Syrup, table blends	1 tablespoon	14.8
Miscellaneous		
Bouillon cubes	2	4.7
Cocoa	2 tablespoons	3.0
Gelatin dessert powder	1 tablespoon	5.3
Beverages		
Beer	12 oz. bottle	12.0
Coca-Cola, ginger ale	8 oz. bottle	21.6
Gin and Rum	1 jigger	0.0
Creme de menthe	1 cordial glass	6.0
Whiskey	—	0.0
Wine, red	1 wine glass	0.5
Wine, port	1 wine glass	4.0

A basic rational diet plan for the obese person would be as follows:

- Sufficient calories to permit physical vigor—approximately 1,100 calories per day for persons engaging in moderate activity, increased to 1,500 calories for greater activity.

- Between 350 and 450 calories per meal, with generous amounts of protein foods.

- Increase in daily exercise.

- Servings of reasonable size; no seconds.

In order to maintain a good caloric control plan the overweight person should take nine steps.

1. Remove visible fat from meat; use only the natural juices, not gravy; broil, boil, or roast meat, fish, and poultry.

2. If low-fat milk is used, corn-oil margarine may be used to flavor vegetables.

3. Steam-cook vegetables, without fat, and add margarine after cooking. This maintains nutrient retention with a low caloric increase. Vegetables can also be flavored with herbs or bouillon cubes.

4. Use low-calorie dressings, vinegar, or lemon on salads.

5. Choose green or yellow vegetables over starchy vegetables like potatoes.

6. Choose fruit desserts over pastries.

7. Sweeten with artificial sweeteners.

8. Schedule meals so that there is a consistent interval between them, thus allowing for proper digestion, assimilation, and excretion.

9. Avoid alcoholic beverages, which are high in "empty"
    calories.

This type of sensible dieting should provide a negative
calorie balance sufficient to create a weight loss of a pound
and a half every two to three weeks. This slow weight loss is
ideal in the sense that it does not place excess stress on the
functioning systems, which may be the case with rapid weight
loss.

Most authorities agree that no one should lose more than
a pound or two per week. Thus, in order to lose a pound a
week, cut down your calories by 3,500. Or exercise enough to
burn 3,500 extra calories per week (the chart on p. 98 indicates
random activities and their attendant calorie consumption).
The best way to lose weight is a combination of both methods,
diet and exercise.

Exercise and Diet

Let us consider an example of this concept. Gymnastics
burn up from 200 to 500 calories per hour. With one hour per
day of this activity at a rate of 200 calories per hour, you must
reduce your calorie intake by only 300 per day to attain the
goal of a pound (3,500 calories) off a week.

The diet should be low in foods containing cholesterol,
such as shellfish, liver, kidneys, and in particular egg yolks,
and also foods that raise the cholesterol count, such as meat,
butter, hard cheeses, cream, whole milk, and chocolate. The
American Heart Association recommends polyunsaturated
foods, which tend to lower blood cholesterol—vegetable oils,
fish, and poultry. An effective and tasty way to reduce cholesterol is to substitute fish and poultry for meat, vegetable oils
for butter, and fat-free milk with the addition of 2 teaspoon-
fuls of unsaturated vegetable oil (soy, safflower, etc.) per
quart for whole milk. Lecithin, a soybean product, has sometimes been shown to be an effective cholesterol reducer when
added to the diet.

In any weight-reduction program we must ensure a balanced diet, one that includes milk, fruits, vegetables, bread, and meat. The average person who wants to take off weight should limit caloric intake to less than 2,700 calories per day. This figure should be adjusted according to the size of the person. In distributing this caloric allowance throughout the day, it is often prudent to allow for some snacks, which yield a certain psychological satisfaction as well as ensuring proper digestion. The less food taken into the stomach at one eating period, the more complete will be digestion and assimilation. Once the ideal weight is secured, the individual should stay within the caloric boundaries of Table 4.5.

If the problem is one of being underweight, reverse tac-

TABLE 4.5
CALORIE ALLOWANCE FOR ADULTS OF AVERAGE
PHYSICAL ACTIVITY

	MEN		
Desirable Weight	25 years	45 years	65 years
110	2300	2050	1750
120	2400	2200	1850
130	2550	2300	1950
140	2700	2450	2050
150	2850	2550	2150
160	3000	2700	2250
170	3100	2800	2350
180	3250	2950	2450
190	3400	3050	2600
	WOMEN		
90	1600	1500	1250
100	1750	1600	1350
110	1900	1700	1450
120	2000	1800	1500
130	2100	1900	1600
140	2250	2050	1700
150	2350	2150	1800
160	2500	2250	1900

tics and increase the weekly intake by 3,500 calories. This should lead to a weekly weight gain of approximately one pound per week. Since either weight reduction or weight gain creates a stress on the body, it is important to lose or gain gradually.

The normal diet should consist of enough calories to maintain normal body weight. Often athletes will not change weight in spite of the rigors of training because their fat weight is being changed to muscle weight. The athletes change the composition of their body, but not their weight. Normally, the individual in training requires approximately 4,000 calories per day. For grammar school or high school athletes this allowance should be adjusted to accommodate the rapid growth rate. On the college level it has been found that a daily diet of 5,000 to 6,000 calories is necessary for football and crew, a bit less for hockey, baseball, and track.

The diet should provide sufficient carbohydrate reserves needed for excess muscular metabolism. Approximate daily dietary requirements are 20 percent protein, for proper growth and repair of tissue; 40 percent carbohydrates, for quick energy reserves; and 40 percent fat, for long-term energy and endurance (fat also acts as a digestive "vehicle" for the fat-soluble vitamins A, D, E, and K). These figures should be adjusted according to type and duration of training and other factors. The eating hours should be regularized to complement training time. Enough time should be allowed to ensure proper digestion and absorption.

The diet should supply plenty of fresh green vegetables, whole-grain flour products, milk and milk products, and animal and vegetable fat—all ensuring an adequate intake of vitamins and minerals.

In most cases the standard three-meals-a-day routine is acceptable. People seem to function better on five meals a day. This must be worked out by the individual. It is a cardinal nutritional sin for those in training to omit breakfast, especially the young athletes. Poor academic and athletic performance can often be traced to the skipping of breakfast. This omission day after day creates deficiencies in the growing athlete that may cause irretrievable encumbrances in sports as one progresses.

As we have established, the general training program is of prime importance if the athlete's to maintain optimal functioning capacity. We now must continue on to individual regimes relating to the needs of specific sports.

5 NUTRITIONAL GUIDELINES FOR SPECIFIC SPORTS

Diet requirements are essentially the same for all sports, but the nutritional needs of some athletes, such as pro-football players and track stars, are naturally greater than those of others, such as the weekend jogger, tennis player, or golfer. Unfortunately, not enough research has been done to outline nutritional data for every athletic endeavor. Perceptive individuals will absorb the following information and tailor it to their own needs.

ENERGY COST OF SPORTS

Different sports require different applications of energy. The more arduous muscular activity is, and the longer it lasts, the greater is the energy used. Energy metabolism becomes more complex as the sport requires more endurance or excessive stress, and so do the nutritional requirements.

Sports may be divided basically into two categories—low-energy cost and high-energy cost. Field events, ski jumping, and diving are considered single efforts, demanding strength and quick reactions, but since they are participated in for less than one hour per day, they demand a low energy rate. Other sports such as golf and archery are also typical of the activities with relatively low energy needs. The demands placed on the body's energy stores are for brief periods only, and so utilization of stored energy is a fraction of that used by sports requiring extra energy expenditure. It is true, however, that low-energy-cost activities can conceivably be termed as high-energy-cost activities if they are carried on intensively for long periods of time. This is exemplified by tennis matches or golf games that are prolonged into grueling competitions for sustained periods.

Some of the short-duration sports—those requiring relatively low energy—are as follows:

Archery	Javelin throw
Baseball	Judo
Basketball	Pole vaulting
Boating	Running (short-distance)
Bowling	Shot-put
Boxing	Skating
Canoeing	Skiing (short-distance)
Cycling	Ski jump
Diving	Softball
Equestrian sports	Sprints
Fencing	Swimming (short-distance)
Golf	Tennis
Gymnastics	Volleyball
High jump	Weight lifting
Hurdle races	

Sports that may be classified as requiring high energy are as follows

Canoeing (long-distance)	Running (long-distance)
Football	Skating (long-distance)
Gymnastics	Skiing (long-distance)
Handball	Skin diving
Ice hockey	Soccer
Field hockey	Swimming (long-distance)
Marathon	Tumbling

Mountaineering   Water polo
Pentathlon   Wrestling
Rowing (long-distance)

Naturally, sports requiring sustained periods of time and great energy expenditure have caloric needs above the ordinary everyday diet. Often the athlete needs to increase his intake up to 4,000 or 5,000 calories per day—depending, of course, on body size and weight. Table 5.1 shows how many calories are expended on some typical athletic activities.

Two widespread misconceptions in this area are that nu-

TABLE 5.1
APPROXIMATE ENERGY COST OF COMMON SPORTS AND EXERCISES

SPORT	CALORIES EXPENDED PER MINUTE OF ACTIVITY
Football	8.9
Running (short-distance)	13.3–16.6
(cross-country)	10.6
Swimming (breast stroke)	11.0
(backstroke)	11.5
(crawl; 50 yards per minute)	14.0
Squash	10.2
Wrestling	14.2
Skiing (moderate speed)	10.8–15.9
(maximum speed)	18.6
Tennis	7.1
Golf	5.0
Cycling (5.5 mph)	4.5
(9.5 mph)	7.0
(13.0 mph)	11.1
Rowing (50 strokes per minute)	4.1
(87 strokes per minute)	7.0
(97 strokes per minute)	11.2
Skating (fast)	11.5

trition does not affect athletic performance and that nutrition is not important. There are many arguments among sports people about pregame meals, vitamins, food supplements, and other factors. However, all intelligent people concede that more information should be gathered and then disseminated to coaches, athletes, and their families.

Professional and collegiate mentors often are narrow in their concerns. At first they tend to believe that training alone is the way to achieve optimum performance. Often, when they later consider diet and nutrition, they tend to go overboard and fall for the faddist or gimmicky approaches. One fact is paramount. There are no easy solutions. Supplementation alone is not the answer. Nor is training.

ADVICE FROM TWO NUTRITION EXPERTS

David G. Guy, Ph.D., is a noted nutritional researcher. In a letter to one of the authors he stressed the growing awareness that the athlete needs additional minerals as well as added vitamins.

There seems to be an increased requirement for zinc, iron, magnesium, and potassium. There also seem to be some indications that the B vitamins and ascorbic acid are needed in larger amounts; however, the data on these particular nutrients are not well substantiated. One might generalize that those vitamins and minerals which are water soluble are needed in larger amounts, probably because of sweat loss.

All nutritionists seem to agree on the need for protein in the diet of the growing athlete. Dr. Guy notes that:

The amount of carbohydrate and fat needed in the diet is a much more complex problem. The preferred source of energy for the muscle is carbohydrate. It appears from the scientific literature that the more the muscle is worked, the higher the demand for carbohydrate. Various Swedish workers have shown that it is possible to increase the level of carbohydrate in the muscle; however, this requires very complex dietary manipulation. The procedure is to work the athlete to exhaustion a week prior to the event, then feed him a high fat–low carbohydrate diet. Two days prior to the event they feed a very high carbohydrate–low fat diet. This diet will consist of nearly 70% of the calories coming from carbohydrate. As you can see, this would meet with very little acceptance to the normal athlete, and indeed this is the case. These workers are continuing to modify their approach for this reason, and I expect within the next several years a definitive answer for the amount of carbohydrate needed in the diet of the athlete will be available.

I might also add to date all the experimental data has been from athletes in endurance events; there is no word available on athletes performing strength events.

Concerning liquid diets for the pregame meal, Dr. Guy says that most of these products contain lactose as the carbohydrate and that "lactose (milk sugar) has come to be recognized as the major reason why many people are not drinking milk or milk-based products. It has been found that 70% of blacks and nearly 90% of the Orientals are unable to consume milk-based products because of lactose intolerance." Naturally, those athletes must select a pregame liquid meal that does not contain a milk-based carbohydrate.

Autti Ahlstrom, D. Sc., acting Associate Professor of Public Health Nutrition at the University of Tampere, Finland, has collected information on the nutritional habits of top Finnish athletes by interviewing them.

TABLE 5.2
PROTEIN INTAKE OF REPRESENTATIVE ATHLETES

	NUMBER OF PERSONS STUDIED	USERS OF PROTEIN PREPA- RATIONS	AVERAGE INTAKE OF PROTEIN FROM FOOD, G/DAY*	INTAKE FROM PROTEIN SUPPLEMENTS, G/DAY†
Hockey players	19	5	166	0.4–2.0
Weight lifters	7	6	210	1.7–21.0
Runners	14	11	168	1.4–4.4

*Measured by 24 hr recall method
†Lowest and highest intake among those using protein supplements

A chart prepared by Dr. Ahlstrom and two associates, P. Ronkainen and L. Peltosaari (1973) graphically explains the limited value of protein supplements to a "bulk" type of athletics such as weight lifting.

Are there marked differences in performances by athletes in response to diet-supplement programs? Dr. Ahlstrom says, "It is the main issue of several coaches (especially track and field) that dietary supplements are one of the reasons or even the main reason for the improvement of performance noted in our top athletes."

The reader can see that nutritional information has become of utmost importance, although the science has lagged behind the demand. As Dr. Ahlstrom explains, "As far as I can tell, the medical attitude has been and still is somewhat cautious in nutritional matters in connection with sports."

Dr. Ahlstrom feels that "No vitamin supplement is necessary in the case of athletes with the possible exception of ascorbic acid, which is known to be quite low in ordinary Finnish diets due to the limited intake of fruits and berries. . . ." He goes on to state that "Basic nutritional facts in simple terms should be taught not only to the athletes but especially to their coaches in order to build a nutrition knowledge strong enough to resist all sorts of foolish ideas and magic concerning nutrition."

Dr. Ahlstrom concludes by stating:

> A good nutritional status is, of course, extremely important to the athlete, and I think it can be achieved by using ordinary well-balanced diets together with reasonable timing of the meals. On the other hand, special nutritional measures are of importance with regard to diets during the days immediately before the competition (high-carbohydrate diet for runners, etc.) as well as during the competition day (light meals). In general the rise in athletic performance can in many cases be attributed to increased exercise together with improved food habits.

ADVICE FROM THE ATHLETES, COACHES, AND TRAINERS

Since many athletic organizations place no particular importance on diet and nutrition, they have not accumulated any data on how diet aids the athlete. A few sports in the last generation have become concerned with the subject. Some coaches and athletes are more concerned with nutrition than are others.

Because of the increased popularity of collegiate and professional football, teams across the country have experimented with diets and pregame meals, liquid diets, and so on. Participants in track events (especially runners) have been interested in nutrition more than other athletes from any other sport activity. Persons involved in karate, judo, weight lifting, and jogging are generally more concerned with the total body, hence are aware of nutritional habits. And because weight control is so important to wrestlers they are also concerned with diet.

Football

Tracy Ladd, Head Trainer for Louisiana State University's football team, says ". . . everyone is hunting for short cuts and surefire ways." Ladd feels that there is an observable difference in the performances of those athletes who maintain a good dietary and supplemental program. "I can see this development during the season." He claims that changes of attitude are occurring in the medical community, and that they are finally killing some old myths.

Ladd feels that vitamin therapy should be used when a deficiency exists, but he is not totally convinced at what point this is reached. He does, however, recommend one therapeutic vitamin formula daily, perhaps two pills during recovery from an illness. He recommends the following diet for the LSU football team:

Early in week—high protein, moderate carbohydrate
End of week—high carbohydrate, low protein
Day of event—almost all carbohydrate
Heavy weights—run, run,—stretch, stretch,
          three days per week

Ladd makes the sound suggestion that education procedures should be instituted in junior high school. He says to young athletes, "Eat smart and balanced meals—stay away from fads and gimmicks. When it is time for you to grow, you will, not before."

Interestingly enough, this experienced trainer feels that injuries may be aided along the road to recovery with "high vitamin C, iron and zinc supplements along with balanced meals."

His advice to youngsters interested in football: "Be patient and smart—you cannot cheat on or push nature—presently we cannot change metabolism, use some common sense."

Running

Ian Jackson, of *Runner's World,* a periodical geared mainly toward track events, appears to be against supplementation of any kind: "Vitamins are catalysts—needed for the full assimilation of foods. They are found in organic combination with other nutritive elements in whole foods—and that is how they should be taken."

He recommends that athletes adopt "a vegetarian or lac-to-vegetarian diet, mainly raw. Avoid anything that has been refined or processed in any way (where the food value is taken out) or that contains additives of any kind (possible toxic products put in)."

Jackson feels that the athlete should learn about the basics—the physiology of nutrition must always be the starting point. "It's not what you eat that nourishes you, but that portion of it that your body can digest and assimilate." He adds that the junior high school or high school athlete should "Mainly give up all junk foods, and give up snacking. I would say 'read, read, read.' The highly motivated youngster will devour anything that can be of use to his athletic progress."

Some respected athletes feel that maintaining a weight below the chart weight is ideal, especially for runners. Ernst van Aaken, a German coach and physician, claims that distance runners should be 20 percent below the average weight for their height, since the greater a runner's heart volume in relation to his body size, the more endurance he has.

Olympic gold medalist Frank Shorter is 5'10½" and 134 pounds, which is exactly 20 percent below the average. On the other hand, Jon Anderson, 1973 Boston Marathon winner and Olympic 10,000-meter man, is 6'2" and 160 pounds, about "chart" weight, which he says is preferable for marathon running. Runner Jeff Galloway agrees with the underweight theory. "I'm convinced you run much better the skinnier you are."

Karate

James Fraracci is the youngest person ever to receive a fourth-degree black belt in karate; he got it when he was 23. He teaches karate and does stunt work in TV and films and is an ardent promoter of health.

He tells us that a superior diet is necessary for his work. He eats meat, fish, eggs, cheese, vegetables, fruits, and natural, unrefined foods. His nutritional interest began when he was 15 years old. At that time he felt it was the road to top performance.

Fraracci's karate students have offered him the opportunity to observe the results of nutrition. "Those that follow a natural diet look better, come to class more, and even perform better." He thinks that current data has shown proof of his convictions.

"Vitamins E, C, and the B complex help," claims Fraracci, "but they are not the panacea. Determination is the most important aspect.

As a believer in vitamins, Jim takes them regularly. His regimen consists of 3,000 milligrams of vitamin C, 1,000 I.U. of vitamin E, and a multi-vitamin-mineral tablet daily. This supplementation along with his aforementioned diet plus liver at least once a week, says Jim, affords him all the nutritional boost he needs to reach his maximum capacity. As far as he is concerned there is no off-season. "I practice karate, jog, and do weight training all year round."

He advises the young athletic aspirant to "read all the available data on nutrition, no smoking, drinking, drugs, and eat natural, unrefined foods with a minimum intake of sugar."

If any injuries occur, Jim depends primarily on the healing power of nature, assisted by a "light fruit diet and vitamin C."

Judo

J. J. Fitzsimmons of the National Judo committee feels that the most popular misconceptions are that a big breakfast and steak on the day of the tournament, and honey just before the tournament, are the roads to success.

Unfortunately, most judo participants are interested in nutrition "only for a few days before 'the big one.' " Fitzsimmons feels that nutrition as related to sports is a concern of only about 30 percent of all athletes. He also claims that the medical attitude toward nutrition is "probably not" changing.

According to Fitzsimmons diets are a matter purely of likes and dislikes, the only stipulation being that one should not compete on an empty stomach. He also maintains that regular workouts should be maintained year round, and that there should be ". . . unbiased, thorough, practical education for everyone."

Outside of a regular balanced diet, Fitzsimmons does not agree with any vitamin-supplement theories, "unless it is required as the psychological boost."

Weight Lifting

Jerry Brainum, a professional body builder and health enthusiast, holds among his titles the following:

1958—AAU Jr. division swimming champion
1966—Mr. North Jersey
1967—Mr. Eastern America
1967—Jr. Mr. East Coast and most muscular
1969—Mr. Central California (3rd)
1969—Mr. Southern California
1974—Mr. Western America (3rd)

Brainum feels that "most coaches and athletes underestimate the value of nutritional supplementation."

Brainum is an avid user of food supplements and recommends them enthusiastically. His college premedical program afforded him a perfect opportunity to investigate this area more than just superficially.

In his mingling with weight lifters and body builders Brainum finds that the two most frequently asked questions are:

1. What are the "energy foods"?
2. What foods help produce strength and stamina?

He feels that there are marked differences in the performance of athletes in response to food-supplement programs, although the medical world has not changed its negative attitude toward this belief.

Brainum feels that athletes should supplement a balanced diet with 800–1,200 I.U. of vitamin E daily along with vitamin-mineral, B-complex, and vitamin C supplements. His suggestions for athletic diets essentially depend on the particular sport, but he feels a general framework of high protein, moderate fat, and low carbohydrate is best.

Unlike many athletes interviewed, Brainum feels that the efficiency of wheat germ oil has been demonstrably proven. He cites the experimentation of Thomas Cureton at the University of Illinois Physical Fitness Lab, who has "tested over 1,000 persons for 10 years." Brainum is a strong believer in wheat germ as a promoter of endurance for athletes.

Brainum agrees that nutritional education should be a "mandatory part of physical education programs in school, by capable, knowledgeable teachers."

Jogging

Jogging has become increasingly popular in the last decade as a method of weight control and as a beneficial exercise—notably for the heart. Here are some tips for the jogger from Dr. T. J. Bassler, editor of the *American Medical Joggers Association Journal.*

> Since we are an organization of physicians who run marathons for prevention of coronary heart attacks we are not primarily interested in racing performances . . . although some of our men do run the 26 miles in well under 3 hours. We are interested in fitness through marathon running.
>
> While we have no standard diet, we do use

about a gram of vitamin C for each 6 miles and
take visible amounts of yeast and wheat germ
oil for their content of B-complex and the unsaturated fats (E.F.A.s). . . .

We do not endorse the use of any specific foods
or diet supplements. Avoiding highly refined foods is
recommended: sucrose, starch, saturated fats and
distilled alcohol. Otherwise a balanced diet with
fresh fruit, raw vegetables, moderate red meat (fish
instead of meat for many meals) plus the wheat
germ oil (or other vegetable oils that are not hy-
drogenated), yeast (or yogurt) and vitamin C (or an
orange for each mile).

Some of our middle-aged men are able to run
5,000–6,000 miles/year on this diet!

Wrestling

Donald L. Cooper, M.D., Director of the Student Hospital
and Clinic at Oklahoma State University, notes,

One thing I have learned in the past few years of
reading, talking, and visiting with literally dozens
of people connected with the sport of wrestling,
especially those who are successful, is that hard
work with a balanced diet, possibly reduced in
quantity but balanced nevertheless, with adequate
fluid intake is the best way to get weight down to
its proper level."

Dr. Cooper also suggests that the wrestler's diet should
be "in the range of 50 percent carbohydrate, 15 to 20 percent protein, and 30 to 35 percent fat. I know it is not
always possible to do this every day, but it is still a worthwhile goal."

TIPS FOR THE ATHLETE

It is appalling that so little concern for diet and nutrition exists in other organized team sports (baseball, hockey, and rugby, for example) or individual pursuits (such as tennis, swimming, bicycling). However, we have compiled some tips for the average athlete.

Present experiments have demonstrated that food taken two to three hours prior to activity has little relevance to energy in short-term events. In events of low-energy cost we suggest that prior to a high carbohydrate pregame diet (begun two or three days before an event) a diet that is mostly fat and protein be maintained.

During high-energy-cost sports a good training diet may include whole-grain bread, meat, eggs and potatoes. A person should also eat liberal amounts of oranges, grapefruit, tomatoes, fresh beans, cabbage, carrots, greens, lettuce, cauliflower, and spinach. These foods are very high in vitamins and minerals, along with the necessary bulk to aid excretion and to avoid constipation.

Supplementation of vitamins A, B, and C provides stimulation of all body secretions and the prevention of nervousness. As far as liquids are concerned, in high-energy-cost activities intake should be in the region of five pints per day, preferably bland liquids.

A high-protein diet that yields about 2,500 calories should be incorporated for high-energy activities until three days prior to an event, generally outlined as in Table 5.3.

It would be best to consult team physicians, dieticians, or nutritionists about specific requirements. If your team or organization does not have a nutritionist or dietician, why not work toward having one? The local chapter of the national organizations of nutritionists and dieticians will probably be happy to make suggestions.

There are several general nutritional guidelines that should be followed by all athletes. After careful study of all available information, we suggest fourteen important rules.

TABLE 5.3
HIGH-PROTEIN DIET FOR ATHLETES IN HIGH-ENERGY SPORTS

FOOD	SERVINGS PER DAY	GRAMS OF PROTEIN
Milk	4 cups	32
Dark-green or yellow vegetables	2 servings	4
Enriched bread and cereal	8 servings	18
Butter, margarine, and fat	7 teaspoons	0
Meat, fish, eggs	10 ounces	35
Fruits and vegetables	2 servings	1
		90

1. Never skip breakfast

2. Eat regularly—five small meals a day is preferable to three heavy meals a day. This aids digestion.

3. Eliminate all junk foods, which provide empty calories (see the snack chart, Table 3.6).

4. Eliminate fatty foods as much as possible before events, because they slow digestion.

5. Eat whole-grain breads or cereals.

6. Eat fortified vegetable oil margarine.

7. Eat fresh fruit every day.

8. Eat four helpings of vegetables every day, especially leaf vegetables and including dark green and yellow vegetables.

9. Drink full fat (or non-fat w/oil added) milk fortified with dry milk solids.

10. Drink a considerable amount of juices and water

11. Keep meals as varied as possible (this will ensure the inclusion of all possible nutrients).

12. Use a caloric, carbohydrate, and protein and fat counter to regularly check on a diet.

13. Athletes should weigh themselves daily. During hot, humid weather water and salts will be lost and must be replaced. The suggestion is one salt tablet taken with one pint of water for every two pounds lost.

14. Experts tend to agree on some supplementation. Russian research has shown that because of stress on the body athletes require additional B-complex and C vitamins (at least double that of the nonathlete). Some coaches and researchers suggest five to ten times more vitamin B-complex and vitamin C for the athlete than the nonathlete. And all seem to agree that vitamin E, wheat germ oil, and wheat germ should be added to the athlete's diet.

Even though there are dietary differences among all sports, and various ideas about food from each player, there is one dietary consideration that is generally agreed upon as being crucially important—the pregame meal. Of course, applying sound nutritional ideas over a long period of time is the ideal, but as in American society in general the immediate-result syndrome is displayed in all sports.

6 THE PREGAME MEAL, LIQUID MEAL, AND OTHER DIETARY CONSIDERATIONS FOR THE ATHLETE

No other chemical compound serves the body so well as does water. The human body is over 60 percent water, while the remaining 40 percent is about 18 percent protein and related substances, 15 percent fat, and 7 percent minerals. People are so dependent on water that if they loses just 10 percent of their supply, they will perish.

Water is the medium in which the chemical reactions of metabolism take place. Water wets the lung surfaces to allow diffusion (movement of carbon dioxide and oxygen) and is important in the uniform distribution of heat and the elimination of excess heat through evaporation. Water is also the transportation system that moves all vital substances through the body. Finally, it serves as a cushion for the spinal column and brain.

The body water may be thought of as all of the water outside the cells, called extracellular fluids (ECF), and all the water inside the cells, or intracellular fluid compartment (ICF).

The amount of water intake required depends on the

temperature of the environment and the amount of physical activity. On a relatively cool day a person engaging in moderate physical activity may lose just 2.5 quarts of water through four major routes—lungs, skin, kidneys, and digestive tract. The same person exercising strenuously on a hot day may lose up to twice that amount.

The normal indicator of water needs is generally thirst. However, most authorities agree that an intake slightly higher than that dictated by thirst is recommended for maintaining maximum kidney health.

Water enters the body in three basic forms: in liquids, in foods, and as a product of oxidation. The obvious main source of water intake is through liquids which supply 1,200 to 1,500 milliliters daily.* The water in foods varies, but the major sources are such "watery" foods as tomatoes, oranges, and watermelon. They provide 700 to 1,000 milliliters daily. The metabolic processes of the body produce water as one result. The amount of metabolic water depends entirely on the nature of the nutrient: for example 100 grams of fat yield 107 grams of water; 100 grams of protein yield 41 grams of water, and 100 grams of carbohydrate yield 55 grams of water. With all forms of water intake considered the body takes in from 2,100 to 2,800 milliliters per day. On the average the body's total output of water is about 2,600 milliliters. The balance of the body's fluids are controlled to a great degree by compounds called *electrolytes*, to a lesser extent by plasma protein, and finally by compounds of small molecular size such as glucose, urea, and amino acids. These latter substances affect water balance only when they occur in unusually large amounts—in diabetes, for example, where an abnormal amount of glucose in the urine causes excess water output.

It is easy to see that water has an important place in athletics. After exercising, a person is thirsty. The first temptation is to satisfy this thirst with large quantities of liquid. This urge should be resisted, and the liquid should be taken

---

*A milliliter is equal to .0338 fluid ounces; 1,500 ml. is a little over 3 pints.

in small amounts over a stretch of time. There is an inevitable lag between the intake of liquid and the following adjustment of the water concentration in the body. During this lag the thirst persists, creating a false need. The free use of water, however, should be allowed during activities, provided it is limited to rinsing of the mouth and swallowing only small sips. Other gimmicks to prevent excess water intake include using a small squeeze bottle or tiny paper cups.

Football and basketball players may lose from 3 to 7 percent of their body weight during competition. This water loss eventually leads to impaired performance. Dehydration should be a consideration as a debilitating factor in any athletic event where body sweat is dominant.

Not only do we lose water during perspiration, we also lose salt. Thus, salt requirements are increased during strenuous activities or when the temperature and/or humidity are excessive. In fact, we recommend moderation of energy output under such conditions. If avoidance is impractical, as is the case with professional athletes, salt tablets, bouillon preparations, or a salt solution of 0.1–0.2 percent concentration is recommended. This solution may be prepared by adding 20 grams of salt to one quart of water, with lemon juice added for palatability. This drink may be given before and after an activity.

Because of the increased muscular activity and water loss through perspiration, the body demands from 7 to 14 ounces of water for every 30 minutes of strenuous activity. This amount is naturally increased if the activity is in a humid, hot environment.

Some authorities claim that the liquid refreshment during athletic activity should be a watery solution of glucose, which has value after an extended period of exertion and competition. This solution replenishes the glucose reservoirs depleted by energy output. Such a drink is especially valuable during long-distance races and endurance events, where an abnormally high amount of sweating occurs. One such solution, Gatorade, was developed by the University of Florida and has become remarkably successful on the commercial market. According to the May 1968 issue of *Science Digest:*

> Researchers have found that football players working out for two hours under Florida's hot September sun lose an average of 7.7 pounds each, most of it through perspiration. When a person drinks water, it must reach what they call "osmotic equilibrium" before the body can absorb it, so trainers and coaches discourage drinking water during strenuous activity.
>
> Now, however, researchers have come up with a solution of water, salts and glucose that closely matches the extra-cellular fluids of the body and is absorbed about 12 times faster than water by means of a process called isotonicity. The scientists have dubbed the beverage they concocted Gatorade. Football players have found they can guzzle a gallon and a half of lemon-lime flavored Gatorade per game.

Another preparation has been developed by J. G. P. Williams, Senior Registrar, Medical Rehabilitation Center (London), for use immediately prior to athletic activity.

1 pint canned orange juice
2 pints drinking water
1 level dessert spoonful (about 8 grains) common table salt
1 level teaspoonful (about 4 grains) bicarbonate of soda
5 grains (.3 gram) soluble aspirin
1 level tablespoonful (approx. 15 grams) powdered glucose

We are assured that this mixture does not violate the doping regulations. We do not agree fully to the use of this mixture, however, particularly with aspirin as an ingredient. Readers may choose for themselves according to their interpretation of all the available information.

Some nitrogen is also lost during heavy or moderate exercise in a hot climate, but this loss is negligible and no extra protein intake is required. This point is reviewed in an article in the *British Journal of Nutrition* (1972).

The Committee of Nutritional Misinformation has prepared a paper, "Water Deprivation and Performance of Athletes," as a statement by the Food and Nutrition Board, Division of Biological Sciences of the National Research Council (May 1974).

Depriving athletes of water has caused avoidable tragedies. Heat stroke, a sudden collapse and loss of consciousness, precipitated by physical exertion and inadequate fluid intake, is a serious hazard during strenuous exercise. Documentary evidence compiled by Dr. C. Blyth in his 1968 report to the American Medical Association on Common Medical Aspects of Sports, spans the years 1961 to 1967. The major predisposing causes of heat stroke cited in this report are high temperature, high humidity, poor body ventilation, and several hours of water deprivation preceding intense physical activity. It is readily apparent that deaths in such cases have occurred because athletic coaches disregarded principles of sound nutrition.

Man can live without food for 30 days, but will die in 5 to 6 days if deprived of water, which is lost constantly. The expired air, urine, sweat and stools remove about 3 pints of water each day from a 70 kg. (154 lb.) individual living in a temperate environment. Optimal physical performance depends upon replacement of water losses.

Water serves as the principal vehicle for transporting substances and heat within the body. In warm environments, it is the only means for dissipating body heat, which is effected by evaporation of sweat. Body heat production is greatly accelerated during physical exercise. Unless water for perspiration is available, the body temperature increases beyond normal and there is overheating. It is imperative that fluid intake be increased to maintain fluid balance as the work level and the environmental temperature increase.

When fluid losses exceed supply, dehydration follows. Excessive fluid loss is almost always accompanied by loss of sodium. In the context of our concern, this is a temporary loss and can be made up by salt intake at the next meal. We are concerned here only with the acute effects of water deprivation. The "dehydration syndrome" is characterized by loss of appetite and limited capacity for work. When there is dehydration, even modest physical activity causes heart rate and body temperature to increase. Physiological changes that impair performance are detectable with losses no greater than 3 percent of the body water. When losses are 5 percent, evidence of heat exhaustion becomes apparent and at 7 percent, hallucinations occur, which is a dangerous sign. Losses totaling 10 percent are extremely hazardous and lead to heat stroke. If not treated immediately, death will result. Heat stroke is accompanied by high body temperature (106–110°F) and deep coma. In most cases there is complete absence of sweating and failure to form urine is common. Convulsions may occur. Immediate medical attention is mandatory.

There is no basis for restricting water intake of athletes during contests nor is there any evidence that man can adapt or be trained to tolerate water intake lower than his daily losses. On the contrary, the scientific literature on the subject strongly supports the practice of replacing water loss by continuous fluid intake. If coaches encourage moderate fluid intake (after acclimatization), light clothing, proper provisions for ventilation, and rest periods, physical

activity which causes profuse sweating can be tolerated even at high temperature.

Deliberate dehydration is never an acceptable
method for control of body weight. It causes temporary loss of weight which is rapidly regained by rehy-
dration. Loss of body weight should occur only at the
expense of body fat, not water or protein. Control of
body weight in normal individuals should be based on
intake and expenditure of calories. When the daily
expenditure of calories exceeds the intake, loss of
body weight occurs. If intake exceeds energy expenditure there is weight gain. Coaches and trainers
frequently require young wrestlers and boxers to
attain specified weights that are considerably below
their usual weight. They have advised youthful athletes to lose body weight by "crash" caloric restriction or by "drying out" for the "early weigh in"
following which they attain their usual weight for
the contest.

These practices can cause permanent impair-
ment of health and even death and have been con-
demned by the American Medical Association.

Athletes should be alerted to the danger of diminished urine volumes which can result in kidney
damage. Urine volume should be maintained at no
less than 900 ml. (one quart) per day.

Summary

Water losses of the body should be replaced by
frequent small intakes of water throughout the day.
Water restriction does not reduce the fluid requirement, but it does impair performance. Dehydration
limits the capacity to work, largely through impaired
cardiovascular function. Death can result if water
loss exceeds 10–20 percent of body water. Unless the
sweat loss is replaced at frequent intervals during
physical activity, heat exhaustion can develop. Ath-

letes and coaches should be aware of the hazards of water deprivation and take steps to avoid excessive dehydration. Body weight control in adolescents either by severe water or caloric restriction is a dangerous practice not to be condoned.

THE LIQUID MEAL

There is much controversy over the benefits of a liquid meal as opposed to a solid-food meal. In the *Journal of the Oklahoma State Medical Association* Dr. Donald L. Cooper, Director of the Student Hospital and Clinic at Oklahoma State University, states:

> For centuries trainers and coaches have advocated special dietary schemes, stemming from older traditions and superstitions, and based on the belief that the ingestion of particular foods would augment the physical capacity or efficiency of the performer.

Dr. Cooper maintains that such beliefs are still part of the athletic scene, especially in college wrestling and boxing, where competitors "frequently resort to crash diets in an attempt to qualify for a lower weight classification, even though they may sacrifice strength and stamina as a result." He goes on to explain that many athletes indulge in health foods, thinking that some magic ingredient may enable them to perform beyond their normal capacity.

Dr. Cooper distills his thoughts as follows:

> "Although relatively little investigation has been done on the special nutritional problems of athletes, the best available evidence today indicates that the athlete performs best on a balanced diet that in-

cludes a high carbohydrate content for quick energy, protein for growth and repair of tissue, ample supplies of vitamins and minerals, and moderate-to-low fat content. In terms of daily caloric requirements, of course, the athlete's needs are considerably higher than those of the average person. In a study of the actual eating habits of athletes at one college, Mays and Scoular calculated that the average football player (mean of 72 inches in height and 198 pounds in weight) consumed 4,600 calories a day during the competitive season and 5,030 calories a day during the preseason training period.

The article continues by noting that sound nutrition is difficult to achieve when coupled with pregame stress. A few years ago researchers who suspected that "vomiting and sluggishness noted in certain football players could be traced to pregame tension, conducted barium X-ray studies on four volunteers who ate the customary big meal four hours before playing a game." The results of the tests showed clearly that the athletes required from two to four hours longer than usual to digest their food than normal young males in a nonstress situation. The researchers concluded from their data that the reason for this was pregame emotional stress reducing gastrointestinal motility rather than any physiological malfunction.

The article continues:

As an outgrowth of this study, the University of Nebraska football team tested a revised pregame feeding schedule throughout the 1960 season. Instead of the usual 1,858 calorie solid breakfast, each player was given a light breakfast of toast, honey and peaches at 9 A.M. the morning of an afternoon game. At 10:30 each player drank one or two glasses of a liquid food which was the equivalent of a nutritionally complete meal. X-rays on volunteers showed that the liquid food passed through the stomach in less than two hours. . . . It did not differ from the conventional solid meal with respect to subsequent hunger, diarrhea, or weight changes, but in those who took it dryness of the mouth was less frequent during the game, strength and endurance seemed to improve, and both vomiting and muscular cramps were eliminated."

Oklahoma State University, claims Dr. Cooper, paid particular attention to this report because their athletes had had more than their usual share of gastrointestinal problems. One-fifth of the squad voluntarily eliminated breakfast on the day of the game after discovering how difficult energy output was with undigested food in the stomach. Dr. Cooper claims that "during preseason practice, when the squad worked out twice a day in summer heat, it was common for eight to twelve boys a day to suffer from dry heaves, vomiting or similar complaints."

During the 1961 season Dr. Cooper conducted an experiment with a popular liquid food product. The product is prepackaged and contains 12½ fluid ounces, providing 400 calories, 20 grams of protein, 50 grams of carbohydrates, and 13.3 grams of fat, along with essential amounts of vitamins and minerals. This product was used throughout preseason training and as a pregame supplement during regular football season. Dr. Cooper concludes from his informal observations that "Impressions were so favorable that we are continuing to use the [liquid meal] and have begun to use it in other sports as well."

THE PREGAME MEAL

Food intake is always important in athletics, but it is crucially important in terms of the pregame meal. There has been a great deal of attention given to this point over the years. In an article in the *Canadian Medical Association Journal* in June 1951 Dr. E. H. Bentley indicates that the most important aspect in considering the food of the athlete is the emotional stress encountered. Stress may cause loss of appetite, abdominal discomfort, and even vomiting or diarrhea. If a meal is consumed too close to the time of the activity, the anxiety of the athlete may impede performance. Therefore, the first principle is not to eat less than three hours before the event. Individual food choices should be respected, since the athletes have probably learned which foods agree or disagree with them. In general, only highly digestible food should be part of the pregame meal.

For strenuous activities the pregame period should start about 48 hours before the event. Some authorities claim that events requiring low-level endurance usually are not affected greatly by eating habits. Prior to competition foods that cause gas should be decreased along with roughage and foods that increase stool bulk. Foods that should be eliminated entirely are oils, spices, salads, alcohol, and rough and seedy vegetables. The foods to be eaten are those that are easily digestible, bland, and nongreasy. Ideally, these foods should be high in carbohydrate content, preferably in liquid form. This allows an adequate glycogen supply for energy and to protect against low blood sugar, which creates a feeling of fatigue. Also, carbon dioxide is the major acid created by the metabolism of carbohydrates, and it can be discharged easily through the lungs and skin. On the other hand, a high protein pregame meal, such as meat and eggs, creates acid that must be handled by the kidneys. During heavy exercise the kidneys have blood forced around them, inhibiting their function of eliminating the metabolic waste of protein assimilation. As a result greater acidosis and fatigue occur than in the metabolism of carbohydrates.

In addition, the excretion of protein metabolic wastes requires an excess water intake, resulting in additional urination. One can imagine how disagreeable this can be.

There is an efficiency factor that gives another point to

carbohydrates. It appears that carbohydrates are 10 percent more efficient in utilizing oxygen than fats or proteins. Five calories are produced as a result of one liter (approximately one quart) of oxygen-burning carbohydrates, whereas only 4.5 calories are produced when an equal amount of oxygen burns fats or proteins.

A recommended pregame meal would consist of a balanced liquid food (commercially or self prepared) along with toast and honey, a soft cereal (oatmeal, cream of rice), weak tea with honey, and soft fruits in syrup (peaches).

The picture is not quite as simple as it may appear. Too many carbohydrates may bring diminishing returns. In the *Journal of the American Medical Association,* Vol. 223 (1973) an article titled "Carbohydrate Loading a Dangerous Practice" reviews intensive studies by Dr. Astrand, a noted physiologist, that raise serious questions as to the advantages of carbohydrate intake. In tests on competitive distance runners Dr. Astrand concluded that carbohydrate "loading" (excess intake of carbohydrates for increased endurance) can lead to cardiac infarction in susceptible individuals.

The majority of authorities and athletes seem to agree that the liquid meal is the ideal solution.

A paper in the *Athletic Journal* (1968) described a survey that was conducted of 48 junior and senior high school males—24 varsity players and 24 seventh and eighth graders. Prior to the study each boy received a physical examination and had his weight recorded. The test covered a ten-week period for the varsity members and six weeks for all the rest. These periods covered practice sessions, nine senior varsity interschool competition games, and six junior team games.

The liquid meal was supplied in 12½-ounce cans containing 375 calories—25 grams of protein, 11 grams of fat, 44 grams of carbohydrate, and the essential vitamins and minerals (there are a few liquid supplements that fit this description closely).

The varsity players ate their regular pregame meal at 2:30 P.M. and had one can of supplement at 5:00 P.M.; the games were at 7:00 P.M. The supplement was again available at halftime. The players drank at least one can immediately after each daily practice and at least one can after dinner.

Records were kept on all of the participants, and results were computed. Their weights were modified acceptably, and they did not become as tired even though the coaching staff was expanded and the practices became more strenuous and better controlled. As a result of the increased conditioning the players became stronger and had fewer injuries. It was also noted that fewer muscular cramps occurred than in previous years. The varsity team had its best season in years, winning the conference. The seventh and eighth graders had an undefeated season, winning their conference.

Many surveys of this type have praised the advantages of the liquid meal. Writing in the *Athletic Journal* (January 1966) Ray Robison, Arizona State trainer, claims that the strenuous regime his athletes follow keeps them from achieving the proper body weight. He says that adding a liquid food supplement to the diet solves the problem. He recommends a can of liquid food with the evening meal and another before retiring. This adds approximately 800 calories to the diet.

The article claims that X-rays have proven that a solid pregame meal is not digested, and therefore produces no energy. The athlete must then depend on reserve energy stores for strength. This leaves even well-conditioned athletes with difficulties on game day.

Robison maintains that liquid pregame meals can be absorbed and converted into playing energy in less than three hours. He feels that athletes who choose a liquid pregame meal have a decided edge over those who choose a solid one. He suggests that each athlete be given a can of liquid nutrition two hours before game time. This provides easy digestion, faster assimilation (and thus quicker energy), and the elimination of problems connected with traveling.

Another advantage to a liquid meal is the convenience on the road. This choice eliminates the difficulty of coordinating meals and all of the attendant disadvantages.

The Arizona State University wrestling team used a liquid food supplement in their nutrition program for one year. This program helped bring the wrestlers down to the proper weight class gradually, without loss of strength and stamina.

In summary, authorities recommend liquid meals for weight gain, for weight loss, and for the pregame meal. If athletes were given the chance to try a liquid meal, odds are that the coaches and trainers would be convinced of its merits and subsequently use it in training programs.

Interest in the pregame meal has always been high, and filled with controversy. Jeff Fair, football trainer at Oklahoma State University, wrote his master's thesis at the University of North Dakota on this theme. He studied 68 Oklahoma State University football players who ran two miles after consuming one of the following four diets:

Steak Precompetition Meal—*approximately 893 calories (20)*
   6 oz. orange juice
   8 oz. steak (med.)
   1 scrambled egg
     plain jello mold (strawberry)
   2 slices dry toast
     hot tea
   2 packets sugar
   2 packets honey
   1 pat of butter

Pancake Precompetition Meal—*approximately 1,889 calories (20)*
   6 oz. orange juice
   4 6″ diameter pancakes—hot syrup (4-oz. ladle)
     plain jello mold (strawberry)
   2 slices dry toast
     hot tea
   2 packets sugar
   2 packets honey

1 glass of milk
3 pats of butter

Oatmeal Precompetition Meal—*approximately 1,062 calories (20)*
6 oz. (bowl) oatmeal
1 scrambled egg
2 slices dry toast
2 glasses of milk
2 pats of butter
2 packets sugar

Control Precompetition Meal—*0 calories*
No food ingested

According to this study the four diets had no effect on performance. The majority of subjects who ate the steak and eggs showed a preference for that meal, and those who chose the other meals preferred them. Jeff concluded on the basis of his questionnaire and the athletes' performances that the psychological factors involved in the pregame meal may be more important than the meal itself.

As a result of these findings Oklahoma State has instituted a spaghetti night on Thursday, in hopes that the added carbohydrate consumption will increase the glycogen supply for the Saturday game.

The following menus have been chosen by Jeff Fair for the university football team's Friday and pregame meals.

Friday: 6:00 P.M.
8 oz. tomato juice (mild)
Chef's salad—(approximately a 12-oz. salad bowl with lettuce, tomatoes, ham, cheese, and a choice of dressing and crackers)
Sirloin strip or T-bone steak (14-oz. steak, cooked medium)
Large baked potato (butter for potato on the table)

Serving of green beans or peas

Plenty of rolls, butter, and honey on the tables

Pitchers of milk on the tables, and choice of another beverage for each person (coffee, iced tea, or Coke)

Pie à la mode (apple, cherry, or blueberry with vanilla ice cream)

Friday: 9:00 P.M.

Milk Shakes (chocolate or vanilla)

Saturday: 10:00 A.M. Brunch

6 oz. orange juice

Fresh citrus fruit cup (oranges, grapefruits, and pineapples)

3 scrambled eggs

4 oz. slice of ham

Hash brown potatoes (nongreasy)

Large breakfast roll or pastry

Buttered toast, honey, jelly, and butter

Choice of beverage (milk, iced tea, hot tea, or coffee)

Steak Pregame Meal (for approximately 40 people)*

6 oz. orange juice

Sirloin strip steak (8 oz. cooked medium)

Baked potato (medium size)

Plain Jello

Platters of dry toast and plenty of honey on the tables

Butter (3 pats per plate)

Pitchers of hot tea on the tables

Choice of another beverage (iced tea or coffee)

Pancake and Small Steak Pregame Meal (for approximately 20 people)

6 oz. orange juice

Sirloin strip steak (4 oz. cooked medium)

*Pregame meals to be served at 3:30 P.M. Saturday

Pancakes (three cakes approximately 6 inches in diameter, each with hot syrup)
Plain Jello
Platters of dry toast and plenty of honey on the tables
Butter (3 pats per plate)
Pitchers of hot tea on the tables
Choice of another beverage (iced tea or coffee)

Pancake Pregame Meal (for approximately 10 people)

6 oz. orange juice
Pancakes (four cakes approximately 6 inches in diameter, each with hot syrup)
Plain Jello
Platters of dry toast and plenty of honey on the tables
Butter (3 pats per plate)
Pitchers of hot tea on the tables
Choice of another beverage (iced tea or coffee)

The liquid nutrients used in the pregame meal should be easily absorbable and low in fat. This is the reason that skim milk is used along with liquids that have a controlled salt content (too little results in low-sodium syndrome, whereas too much precipitates thirst)

The following liquids can be used by the athlete if they do not cause any discomfort:

Skim milk
Lemonade
Limeade
Apple juice
Clear chicken
   and beef broth
Bouillon
Consummé
Diluted orange and pineapple juice

We feel in all cases both tea and coffee should be eliminated. The caffeine in either of them overstimulates the central nervous system in the athlete who is already stimulated by the excitement of the event. There are, however, those coaches and athletes who disagree with this point.

There should also be a decrease in bulk food, which can temporarily eliminate bowel movements that would inhibit athletic performance. For a 48-hour period prior to events the following foods should be eliminated:

Raw fruits except oranges, peeled apple, bananas
Raw vegetables (except lettuce)
Vegetables with seeds
Whole-grain products
Relishes, popcorn, nuts
Jams, preserves
Gravy

Excess amounts of dextrose, glucose, sugar candy, and honey tend to draw too much fluid into the gastrointestinal tract from other parts of the body, thereby causing a dehydration problem that may affect performance.

In many cases the body reacts adversely when the athlete takes in too much sugar. It may also cause stomach distention, and the evacuation mechanism may be impaired. The small intestine may react with cramps, distention, and diarrhea. Any excess carbohydrates can precipitate fermentive activity of intestinal bacteria, which in turn creates gas and diarrhea. Problems of this nature are more likely to occur when the sugars are taken in large amounts of glucose and dextrins.

Postgame foods should be considered as well as those eaten before the event. Since the body takes time to return to normal after an event, it usually does not require much food. Naturally, an athlete should be in a relaxed state when eating, and therefore should wait until the event "jitters" have disappeared. Until this occurs only fruit juices or light fruits should be consumed. When the appetite does return, the athlete should consume a well-balanced meal containing between 500 and 1,000 calories.

It has been found that swimming the 100-yard sprint raises the metabolic rate 10 to 50 times. Even though the energy reserves of a well-developed and properly nourished individual are adequate for strenuous exercises of short duration, there are some who say that even in short-duration exercise the amount of potential work is equated to the amount of food eaten before the event. One successful Olympic athlete says he ingests some dextrose an hour before an event. According to him this extra energy enables him to swim faster and with decreased fatigue. This formula of extra sugar just prior to an event is endorsed by many coaches and athletes. In high-energy sports, of course, the dextrose energy would surely not sustain the participant for extended periods of time.

Another aspect of this subject is discussed in a letter to the editor of *Journal of the American Medical Association* (1972, vol. 222) by Dr. Richard Casdorph and Dr. William Conner, who are doing intensive research on the diet of the Tarahumara Indians of northern Mexico. The men of this tribe are allegedly the world's greatest endurance runners. These Indians live in the caves of the Sierra Madre Mountains at altitudes up to 7,000 feet. They have a kickball game in which competing teams run continuously for 100 to 200 miles. The duration of the competition is from 24 to 48 hours or more, depending on the length of the course.

Essentially the Indians are vegetarians, deriving most of their calories from corn and beans. They supplement this diet with a variety of vegetables and fruits. Occasionally an egg will be eaten, and about once or twice a year, as part of a festival, goat meat will be ingested. Thus, these Indians, who live on a high-carbohydrate diet, are capable of high-level endurance and energy competition. The researchers suggest that long-term ingestion of a high-carbohydrate diet is an effective way to build up glycogen stores for athletic competi-

tion. The researchers also discovered that the serum cholesterol levels of the Indians were strikingly low by the standards of Western Europe and America.)

When considering examples like the preceding, one must
take into consideration the socioeconomic conditions under
which the people lives. It is hardly fair to compare such an
isolated, evenly distributed cultural pattern with our high-
stress social situations. This example merely points out nutritional effects under ideal conditions. They serve to illustrate
that they do exist.

In brief summary we can say that the pregame meal and
diet involve both physiological and psychological considerations. Ultimately, as nutritionist/chemist Dr. Roger Williams
may suggest, one's performance is directly related to biological and psychological individuality. It is the cooperative responsibility of both athletes and their advisors to determine
each individual's diet for maximum athletic performance. This
can be accomplished by investigation, trial, and error.

7 DRUGS AND ATHLETICS

The three "drugs" most widely used by Americans are alcohol, nicotine, and caffeine. These substances are used by people most often because of bad habits rather than as calculated stimulants to prepare for an event or game. In fact, most people in America misuse one of these three.

The generally accepted view is that people in athletics do not smoke or drink. It seems foolish for anyone interested in physical well-being to indulge in such harmful habits as these. Yet, there are many instances of misuse.

ALCOHOL

One of the most widely used drugs today is alcohol in all its forms. Within less than an hour it is absorbed, from the stomach and small intestine into the bloodstream. One gram of alcohol yields seven calories.

Although alcohol affects all the cells of the body, its most dramatic effects are on the brain. Although it is considered a stimulant, it is in fact a depressant to the central nervous system. Loss of integrating control of the cerebral cortex is a result of alcohol's decreasing the inhibitory control mechanism.

It has been indicated that in cases of excessive athletic exertion, alcohol has been administered to athletes as a stimulant, to release inhibitions and decrease fatigue. Findings such as this indicate that the effects of alcohol are primarily on the mind.

In "Drugs in Sports" (1970) Dr. Max Novich offered evidence that European athletes at the turn of the century used alcohol extensively. There were reports of cyclists in 24-hour races drinking rum and champagne throughout the race, of marathon runners and walkers consuming considerable quantities of cognac or beer during competition. Supposedly alcohol had a refreshing effect and the ability to restore the athletes' strength. There are other reports, however, that described how anxiety may develop in the athlete as a result of excessive arousal of the cerebral cortex. Alcohol was termed a doping agent by the International Olympic Committee, but oddly enough it was not listed as such for the '72 Munich Olympics.

There is speculation that alcohol in small quantities may be termed ergogenic in the sense that it inhibits psychological factors that may ordinarily limit performance. On the other hand, studies have demonstrated that motor performance is impaired at low and moderate blood alcohol levels, as are reflexive control and neuromuscular coordination. In sports requiring highly coordinated skills alcohol decreases efficiency.

Current studies have concluded that alcohol also impairs hand-and-eye coordination, complex coordination, balance, and visual tracking.

Since the chronic ingestion of alcohol affects the liver, the organ that resynthesizes glycogen from lactic acid during exercise, higher blood lactate levels may accumulate during exercise. As was noted earlier in this book, the greater the amount of lactic acid, the greater the development of fatigue and consequently impaired performance. Alcohol also exerts deteriorative effects on heart components, thereby conceivably hampering oxygen consumption and decreasing cardiac output.

Because of the widespread social use of alcohol, athletes sometimes fail to see how destructive and debilitating this drug can be. The best advice is to eliminate the use of alcohol except on rare occasions.

NICOTINE

According to the *American Journal of Pharmacy* (1972), nicotine is considered a doping agent. It is a volatile alkaloid derived from tobacco. Small doses of it behave as a stimulant on the central and sympathetic nervous systems in a manner similar to that of amphetamines. In connection with athletics it increases adrenalin secretions from the adrenal medulla, which in turn activates energy output.

Certain research data has indicated that nicotine may also elevate blood sugar levels. Thus, in effect, nicotine alters athletic performance.

A filter cigarette contains 20 to 30 milligrams of nicotine, and the smoker inhales about 10 percent of this amount. Tests have shown that 60 milligrams of nicotine constitutes a fatal dosage. Therefore, it is logical to assume that there is an effect on the body to one degree or another.

CAFFEINE

A popular stimulant that fits into the definition of drug is caffeine. It is a stimulant to the CNS, affecting the cerebral cortex, medulla oblongata, and spinal cord. As a result of this stimulation, wakefulness and mental activity are increased. According to researchers caffeine also stimulates the cardiac muscle and increases the respiratory rate. Caffeine is a natural component of coffee, tea, and cacao beans, and is also available in tablet form. A cup of coffee may contain up to 150 milligrams, and tea and cola drinks may contain half as much. Certain stay-awake commercial compounds contain 110 milligrams per tablet. A normal therapeutic dose of caffeine is 100 to 300 mg.

Valid research has indicated that caffeine may augment the natural release of adrenalin during exercise, thereby possibly producing a potentiating effect. Because caffeine is a natural component of many foods, there is much controversy over whether or not it should be considered a drug. In 1962, the *International Federation of Sports Medicine* undertook a research project dealing with Italian athletes and discovered that caffeine was the most predominantly used "doping" agent. Its use was subsequently forbidden in conjunction with athletic competition. No evidence has been found to suggest that it should be banned by the NCAA, AAU, or IAAF, and it was withdrawn from the doping list of the International Olympic Committee prior to 1972.

The problem of caffeine in relation to hazardous drug abuse is slight. We feel that if athletes choose to drink coffee, tea, or cola drinks, they may do so. If their intake exceeds normal amounts as they try to increase physical capacity, it becomes a problem of greater complexity that must be coped with by the individual's conscience.

"DOPING"

The common everyday drugs should be avoided, but the real problem with drugs and sports is the use of stimulants to enhance performance, steroids to increase growth, and depressants to relax the body. The use of these drugs is referred to in the athletic community as doping. According to the International Congress of Sport Sciences in 1964,

Doping is the administration to, or the use by, a healthy individual of an agent foreign to the organism by whatsoever route introduced, or of physiological substances in abnormal quantities or introduced by an abnormal route with the sole object of increasing artificially and in an unfair manner the performance of that subject while participating in a

TABLE 7.1
DRUGS

Official Name	Slang Name(s)	Usual Single Adult Dose	Duration of Action (Hours)	Method of Taking	Legitimate Medical Uses (Present and Projected)
ALCOHOL Whisky, gin, beer, wine	Booze Hooch Suds	1½ oz. gin or whisky 12 oz. beer	2–4	Swallowing liquid	Rare, Sometimes used as a sedative (for tension).
CAFFEINE Coffee, tea, Coca-Cola No-Doz, APC	Java	1–2 cups 1 bottle 5 mg.	2–4	Swallowing liquid	Mild stimulant. Treatment of some forms of coma.
NICOTINE (and coal tar) Cigarettes, cigars	Fags, Nails	1–2 cigarettes	1–2	Smoking (inhalation)	None (used as an insecticide).
SEDATIVES Alcohol—see above Barbiturates Amytal Nembutal Seconal Phenobarbital Doriden (Glutethimide) Chloral hydrate Miltown, Equanil (Meprobamate)	Downers Barbs Blue Devils Yellow jackets, Dolls Red devils Phennies Goofers	50–100 mg. 500 mg. 500 mg. 400 mg.	4	Swallowing pills or capsules	Treatment of insomnia and tension. Induction of anesthesia.
STIMULANTS Caffeine—see above Nicotine—see above Amphetamines Benzedrine Methedrine Dexedrine Preludin Cocaine	Uppers Pep Pills, Wake-ups Bennies, cartwheels Crystal, speed, Meth Dexies or Xmas trees (spansules) Coke, snow	2.5–5.0 mg. Variable	4	Swallowing pills, capsules or injecting in vein. Sniffing or injecting.	Treatment of obesity, narcolepsy, fatigue, depression. Anesthesia of the eye and throat.
TRANQUILIZERS Librium (Chlordiazepoxide) Phenothiazines Thorazine Compazine Stelazine Reserpine (Rauwolfia)		5–10 mg. 10–25 mg. 10 mg. 2 mg. 1 mg.	4–6	Swallowing pills or capsules	Treatment of anxiety, tension, alcoholism, neurosis, psychosis, psychosomatic disorders and vomiting.
MARIJUANA Cannabis Sativa (5)	Pot, grass, tea, weed, stuff, hash, joint, reefers	Variable—1 cigarette or pipe, or 1 drink or cake (India)	4	Smoking (inhalation) Swallowing	Treatment of depression, tension, loss of appetite, and high blood pressure.
NARCOTICS (opiates, analgesics) Opium Heroin Morphine Codeine Percodan Demerol Methadone Cough syrups (Cheracol, Hycodan, Romilar, etc.)	Op Horse, H, Smack, Shit, Junk Dolly	10–12 "pipes" (Asia) Variable—bag or paper w. 5–10% heroin 15 mg. 30 mg. 1 tablet 50–100 mg. 2–4 oz. (for euphoria)	4	Smoking (inhalation) Injecting in muscle or vein. Swallowing	Treatment of severe pain, diarrhea, and cough.
HALLUCINOGENS LSD Psilocybin S.T.P. D.M.T. Mescaline (Peyote)	Acid, sugar cubes, trip Mushrooms Cactus	150 micrograms 25 mg. 5 mg. 350 mg.	10–12 6– 8 12–14	Swallowing liquid, capsule, pill (or sugar cube) Smoking Chewing plant	Experimental study of mind and brain function. Enhancement of creativity and problem solving. Treatment of alcoholism, mental illness, and the dying person. (Chemical warfare)
ANTIDEPRESSANTS Ritalin Dibenzapines (Tofranil, Elavil) MAO inhibitors (Nardil, Parnate)		10 mg. 25 mg., 10 mg. 15 mg., 10 mg.	4–6	Swallowing pills or capsules	Treatment of moderate to severe depression.
MISCELLANEOUS Glue, gasoline & solvents Amyl nitrite Antihistaminics Nutmeg Nonprescription "sedatives" (Compoz) Catnip Nitrous Oxide		Variable 1–2 ampules 25–50 mg. Variable	2	Inhalation Swallowing	None except for antihistamines used for allergy and amyl nitrite for fainting.

	POTENTIAL FOR						
cho-cal idence	Tolerance (leading to increased dosage)	Physical Dependence	Overall Abuse and Toxicity (2)	Reasons drug is sought (drug effects and social factors)	Short term effects (psychological, pharmacological, social) (3)	Long term effects (psychological, pharmacological, social)	Form of legal regulation and control (4)
gh	Yes	Yes	High	To relax. To escape from tensions, problems and inhibitions. To get "high" (euphoria). Seeking manhood or rebelling (particularly those under 21). Social custom and conformity. Massive advertising and promotion. Ready availability.	CNS (6) depressant. Relaxation (sedation). Euphoria. Drowsiness. Impaired judgment, reaction time, coordination and emotional control. Frequent aggressive behavior and driving accidents.	Diversion of energy and money from more creative and productive pursuits. Habituation. Possible obesity with chronic excessive use. Irreversible damage to brain and liver, addiction with severe withdrawal illness. (D.T.s) with heavy use. Many deaths.	Available and advertised without limitation in many forms with only minimal regulation by age (21, or 18), hours of sale, location, taxation, ban on bootlegging and driving laws. Some "black market" for those under age and those evading taxes. Minimal penalties.
erate	Yes	No	Very Minimal	For a "pick-up" or stimulation. "Taking a Break". Social custom and low cost. Advertising. Ready availability.	CNS (6) stimulant. Increased alertness. Reduction of fatigue.	Sometimes insomnia, restlessness, or gastric irritation. Habituation.	Available and advertised without limit with no regulation for children or adults.
gh	Yes	No	High	For a "pick-up" or stimulation. "Taking a Break". Social custom. Advertising. Ready availability.	CNS stimulant. Relaxation (or distraction) from the process of smoking.	Lung (and other) cancer, heart and blood vessel disease, cough, etc. Higher infant mortality. Many deaths. Habituation. Diversion of energy and money. Air pollution. Fire.	Available and advertised without limit with only minimal regulation by age, taxation, and labeling of packages.
gh	Yes	Yes	High	To relax or sleep. To get "high" (euphoria). Widely prescribed by physicians, both for specific and nonspecific complaints. General climate encouraging taking pills for everything.	CNS depressants. Sleep induction. Relaxation (sedation). Sometimes euphoria. Drowsiness. Impaired judgment, reaction time, coordination and emotional control. Relief of anxiety-tension. Muscle relaxation.	Irritability, weight loss, addiction with severe withdrawal illness (like D.T.s). Diversion of energy and money. Habituation, addiction.	Available in large amounts by ordinary medical prescription which can be repeatedly refilled or can be obtained from more than one physician. Widely advertised & "detailed" to M.D.s & pharmacists. Other manufacture, sale or possession prohibited under federal drug abuse & similar state (dangerous) drug laws. Moderate penalties. Widespread illicit traffic.
igh	Yes	No	High	For stimulation and relief of fatigue. To get "high" (euphoria). General climate encouraging taking pills for everything.	CNS stimulants. Increased alertness, reduction of fatigue, loss of appetite, insomnia, often euphoria.	Restlessness, irritability, weight loss, toxic psychosis (mainly paranoid). Diversion of energy and money. Habituation. Extreme irritability, toxic psychosis.	Amphetamines, same as Sedatives above. Cocaine, same as Narcotics below.
nimal	No	No	Minimal	Medical (including psychiatric) treatment of anxiety or tension states, alcoholism, psychoses, and other disorders.	Selective CNS depressants. Relaxation, relief of anxiety-tension. Suppression of hallucinations or delusions, improved functioning.	Sometime drowsiness, dryness of mouth, blurring of vision, skin rash, tremor. Occasionally jaundice, agranulocytosis, or death.	Same as Sedatives above, except not usually included under the special federal or state drug laws. Negligible illicit traffic.
derate	No	No	Minimal to Moderate	To get "high" (euphoria). As an escape. To relax. To socialize. To conform to various subcultures which sanction its use. For rebellion. Attraction of behavior labeled as deviant. Availability.	Relaxation, euphoria, increased appetite, some alteration of time perception, possible impairment of judgment and coordination. Mixed CNS depressant-stimulant.	Usually none. Possible diversion of energy and money. Habituation. Occasional acute panic reactions.	Unavailable (although permissible) for ordinary medical prescription. Possession, sale, and cultivation prohibited by state narcotic or marijuana laws. Severe penalties. Widespread illicit traffic.
igh	Yes	Yes	High	To get "high" (euphoria). As an escape. To avoid withdrawal symptoms. As a substitute for aggressive and sexual drives which cause anxiety. To conform to various subcultures which sanction use. For rebellion.	CNS depressants. Sedation, euphoria, relief of pain, impaired intellectual functioning and coordination.	Constipation, loss of appetite and weight, temporary impotency or sterility. Habituation, addiction with unpleasant and painful withdrawal illness.	Available (except heroin) by special (narcotics) medical prescriptions. Some available by ordinary prescription or over-the-counter. Other manufacture, sale, or possession prohibited under state and federal narcotics laws. Severe penalties. Extensive illicit traffic.
nimal	Yes (rare)	No	Moderate	Curiosity created by recent widespread publicity. Seeking for meaning and consciousness-expansion. Rebellion. Attraction of behavior recently labeled as deviant. Availability.	Production of visual imagery, increased sensory awareness, anxiety, nausea, impaired coordination; sometimes consciousness-expansion.	Usually none. Sometimes precipitates or intensifies an already existing psychosis; more commonly can produce a panic reaction.	Available only to a few medical researchers (or to members of the Native American Church). Other manufacture, sale, or possession prohibited by state dangerous drug or federal drug abuse laws. Moderate penalties. Extensive illicit traffic.
nimal	No	No	Minimal	Medical (including psychiatric) treatment of depression.	Relief of depression (elevation of mood), stimulation.	Basically the same as Tranquilizers above.	Same as Tranquilizers above.
imal to derate	Not known	No	Moderate to High	Curiosity. To get "high" (euphoria). Thrill seeking. Ready availability.	When used for mind-altering generally produces a "high" (euphoria) with impaired coordination and judgment.	Variable—some of the substances can seriously damage the liver or kidney and some produce hallucinations.	Generally easily available. Some require prescriptions. In several states glue banned for those under 21.

competition. Where the administration of preparations is part of a necessary medical treatment it is
alone the attending physician who may decide in exceptional cases on the individual's ability to participate in a competition. Where the treatment is by
substances, which by their nature, doses and application are able to boost the performance of the athlete
in competition in an artificial and unfair manner, this
is to be regarded as doping and automatically exclud-
ing the ability to compete. In a list to be kept up-to-
date continuously, all those substances were en-
tered, which are in every case to be regarded as
impermissible doping medication. In principle these
include all drugs, weckamines, analeptics, cardiac
medication, respirotonics, psycho-pharmaceuticals,
different alkaloids and hormones.

This commission also felt that extreme suggestive methods such as hypnosis should be categorized as doping. The
athlete, they stated, is reduced simply to a muscle-reflex ma-
chine as a result of hypnosis inhibiting free will and personality.

Even a person with just a slight interest in athletics real-
izes, through the mass media, how extensive drug abuse is
among high school, college, and professional athletes. Unfortunately, most debates on this subject are held in emotionally
charged atmospheres, and only rarely is any clear light shed
upon the matter. In this section we will attempt to share with
the reader as objectively as possible all the information we
have gathered. We are not so presumptuous as to think that
we have solutions to this complex problem. Our aim is to make
the reader aware of the problem, which is in a sense the first
step toward its correction. Of course, the use of drugs as
treatments for illness or injury is not included in our definition
of "doping."

The problem of doping was evident even in ancient Rome,
according to an article in the *Journal of American Veteri-
nary Medical Association.* The Romans gave their horses

hydromel, a mixture of honey and water that increased their endurance and speed during cart races. For hundreds or perhaps thousands of years Indian tribes in Central America have chewed coca leaves to help them in long and arduous mountain journeys. A stimulant contained in the leaves increases endurance and decreases weariness.

In modern times, especially in America and Western Europe, sports are so commercial that there is an exaggerated emphasis on winning. This social pressure forces many athletes and even some trainers to seek out shortcuts to the extra degree of superior performance. Drugs also have an analgesic quality. In sports events that entail many bruises and grueling competition they offer a cushion against pain. Thus, drugs have offered a convenient option, but the problem has gotten out of hand.

In 1960, during an Olympic road race, a young Danish cyclist collapsed and later died as a result of an excessive dose of stimulant. After harsh outcries from various groups, the Danish trainer admitted to having administered beta-pyridyl carbinol, a drug used to increase peripheral circulation. Time and time again there are reports of athletes dying as a result of amphetamine, barbiturate, or even heroin poisoning.

Drugs constitute grounds for disqualification by the U.S. Amateur Athletic Union, the International Amateur Athletic Federation, and the United States Olympic Association.

The most obvious argument against drug abuse by athletes is the danger of physical or psychological harm. We feel that the reason should be more within the fundamental definition of what sport is, the matching of strength and control between competitors based on their natural capacities. The doping of athletes is analogous to cheating at card games. Where is the sport? It merely degenerates into a contest to see which athlete uses the cleverest means of artificial stimulation, and ultimately the athlete cheats himself through self-deception.

As you may have concluded, the definition of drugs is usually rather vague, encompassing anything that alters the normal functioning capacity of the athlete. One might easily fit vitamins or simple glucose into this definition; reducing it to the absurd, we might include even cheering, which motivates the athlete beyond ordinary capacity through hormonal releases and psychological boosts. We think it fair to say that we are concerned with essentially the type of drug that to some extent is detrimental to the body. Of special concern are those drugs that have disastrous side effects such as addiction. This definition can be altered to include even drugs that are *suspect*, such as the anabolic steroids, which increase muscularity but are possible causes of testicular atrophy, prostate cancer, and baldness. (We discuss the steroids later in this chapter.)

Much of Western society has become preoccupied with drug use. It is no longer true that only the sick use drugs. Healthy individuals are using a variety of substances to achieve various effects, to alter personality, or as a key to social interaction. This prevailing social attitude has touched the athlete as well as everyone else. Think of how the slightest variation from the normal pattern causes the healthy middle-class suburbanite to run for a tranquilizer or other mood-altering drug to change the pattern. How much more overwhelming the pressure must be on a professional or amateur athlete in preparation for or during a game! We feel that it would be well to analyze our own consciences in relation to these facts. During these times of instant pleasure at the drop of a pill, it is difficult to condemn the athlete without first condemning the entire society and the circumstances leading to this situation. Our point of view is one of fact presentation, not condemnation or moralizing.

Ostensibly athletes take stimulant drugs to ward off fatigue and to keep up endurance. The body's internal urge to stop activity is in conflict with the external demands of the sport to continue. Herein lies the fundamental physio-psychomotivation to decrease fatigue by any available means. When looked at from the point of view of a drug-oriented culture, the logical step would be—drugs.

The first question is, What is fatigue? Most important, it is the result of excessive muscular exertion, and is attended by alteration in the functioning of the organism. These changes are reflected in increases in perspiration and blood pressure and in a decrease in muscular power.

Muscular exertion brings about an increase of the metabolic processes in the muscle. To fuel this activity the body draws in the amount of oxygen necessary for the utilization of the nutrients available, especially sugar. Carbonic acid is produced as a combustion product and eliminated by the body. When physical exertion depletes the energy stores of the body, an incomplete combustion of glucose occurs. Now, not only is carbonic acid produced but also lactic acid. The latter cannot be removed by the organs of elimination, and so must be combusted further when there is an adequate supply of oxygen.

This state of incomplete combustion creates what is called an oxygen debt, which is paid back by deep and frequent breathing and panting. The production of lactic acid in turn creates an increase in blood and tissue fluid acidity. This condition is known as metabolic acidosis, and it is the prime originator of fatigue. The fatigue syndrome is a body device used to warn athletes that they have reached the limits of their capacity.

Ergogenic Aids

Drugs are used to overcome the physiologic factors of fatigue, such as metabolic acidosis, and also the psychological factors. The most prevalent group of "aids" used by athletes are called ergogenic aids, which are anything that increases energy or energy output. Athletes have always used some ergogenic aid to maximize performance and endurance. These aids may be mechanical or pharmacological in nature. The following substances have been used for a long time and are still being used:

Alcohol	Lecithin
Alkalies	Massage
Amphetamine and other	Mental pictures
sympathomimetic drugs	Negatively ionized air

Anabolic steroids	Oxygen
Caffeine	Peripheral vasodilators
Cardiovascular stimulants	Protein supplements
Cold applications	Salt
Glucose formulas	Ultraviolet rays
Heat applications	Vitamin and mineral supple-
Hormones	ments
Hypnosis	Wheat germ oil

It is obvious to the reader that not all of these aids fall into the category of drug. There is little controversy over many of these aids, and a great deal over the others. The main debate is over the pharmacological ergogenics. As ethical, legal, and moral controversies have grown around these substances, a great deal of research has been done. It is no secret that from the beginning of this century marathon runners, boxers, cyclists, baseball and soccer players, Olympic contestants, and other athletes have used a number of pharmacological agents as ergogenic aids.

Prizefighters of eras gone by were given strychnine tablets, sips of dilute solution of aromatic spirits of ammonia, and drinks of honey and brandy in combination or brandy alone before a fight and between rounds, especially near the end of the bout. Other boxers had their face, neck, and head sponged with champagne to pep them up. Still others were massaged by their trainer with a concoction containing cocaine and coca butter, which offered an anesthetic effect and decreased the pain of the opponent's blows and jabs. Contemporary boxers have notoriously been the victims of schemes involving persons purposely dropping stimulants or barbiturates into their drinking water.

European cyclists use drugs and other substances to withstand the grueling nature of their sport. In fact, many bikers talk openly of their ergogenic aids. French bikers have displayed a preparation known as "caffeine houdes," which are pellets taken for tonic purposes. Another French liquid tonic, "horse blood serum," was packed in 2-cc. ampules and poured into juices or broth just before competition. Belgian riders have been fond of sugar cubes wetted down with a few drops of ether, which they held between the teeth and sucked during the race. Canadian and American riders have had their ergogenic aids as well.

Many six-day bikers have used ordinary caffeine tablets to ward off fatigue. At the beginning of a rest period some riders would take drinks of brandy, beer, or bourbon to make them sleepy. One famous French cyclist slept in an oxygen tent during his rest periods.

Cycle sprinters have also used such aids as nitroglycerin capsules, caffeine capsules, and strychnine. In many cases, heroin and cocaine were given to the riders by their trainers. In fact, cocaine was the most widely used stimulant for professional cyclists. Tight controls have eliminated most of the overt doping of cyclists, but raids still occur in countries like Belgium, France, and Switzerland where six-day races persist.

In recent times, the most popular ergogenic aids have been amphetamines ("uppers") and their derivatives. During the 1930s here benzedrine inhalers were used by American college students to create a state of wakefulness and alertness that allegedly improved athletic performance. During the Second World War uppers were used by soldiers of Allied, German, and Japanese forces to retard fatigue and to produce a feeling of exhilaration before dangerous missions.

After the war, as veterans returned to college, the use of amphetamines spread ferociously as aids to increased stamina and endurance during athletics. Since high school athletes are generally influenced by the activities of college athletes, the use of uppers spread to every level of interscholastic activity.

In *Sports Illustrated* (1959) an article gave the results of amphetamine testing on college athletes at Harvard and at Springfield colleges. "Researchers find that in approximately three-quarters of the cases tested the administration of amphetamines improved performances in weight throwers as much as 3%, in runners as much as 1½%, and in swimmers from .5% to 1.16%."

These results were discussed and analyzed by many who concluded that the uppers did not really improve performance, but merely controlled the fatigue factor or gave a psychological lift. In fact, most of the other tests on performance found no advantages to the use of amphetamines. Ultimately these drugs lead to addiction with all of its dreaded effects.

Extent of the Problem

Although drug abuse is greater on the college and professional levels, evidence shows that the increase on the high school level is appalling. Even athletes of ages 13, 14, and 15 years old are involved. In the April 1972 issue of the *Journal of Health, Physical Education and Recreation*, in an article on "The Realities of Drug Abuse in High School Athletics," Richard Keelor, Director of Athletics at Beverly Hills High, stated that while many coaches and athletic supervisors admit that there is a drug problem, few admit that it is on the high school level. These disbelievers, the article states, feel that the athlete is somehow protected from the drug culture pressure by a "charismatic shield." But if a drug problem exists in the community, chances are that it has infiltrated high school athletics.

High school athletes naturally have idols on the professional and college levels whom they imitate. If they feel their heroes are using stimulants to alter their functioning capacity, they will mimic that action.

In addition to this type of hero imitation, the high school athlete is under a great deal of pressure from coaches, community, parents, and friends to win. Since these pressures are difficult enough to cope with for older, more mature athletes, imagine how much more trying they are for the younger athletes.

There are many testimonies to the extent of high school drug abuse. *Today's Health* magazine in October 1970 ran the results of a survey they took among many people in the sports world on this subject. UCLA team physician Dr. Martin Blazine said "The high school athlete is our greatest concern. Drug abuse has spread to athletes as young as 14 and 15." In the same article Al Silverman, then editor of *Sport*, remarked, "We get reports that 'turning on' with bennies [benzedrine, an amphetamine] is common among high school athletes. It's more far-reaching than most people realize, especially in Texas and Pennsylvania where high school sports are big."

Robert J. Murphy, Ohio State team physician, has received a number of calls from schoolboys and their parents, inquiring about the safety of diet pills (amphetamines that suppress the appetite) for athletes. "The biggest problem," says Dr. Murphy, "are the kids who hear about drugs that improve performance. If one superb athlete takes a drug, word of it often brushfires through the world of sports."

The California State Superintendent of Public Institutions gets "distressing reports about athletes being pepped up or calmed down by drugs." As a research project, a California athlete learned that 48 percent of the players acknowledged having taken uppers at one time or another.

O. J. Simpson, Heisman Trophy winner says, "I don't care what anybody says, in football there are players *on* just about everything. I've seen them taking bennies and stuff like that to get up for a game."

Many times in the current history of sports, doctors have been called on to treat comas and convulsions as a result of drug overdose.

Baseball, the All-American sport, also has its share of drug abuse. In his book *Ball Four*, former Yankee pitcher Jim Bouton claims that "A lot of players need 'greenies' just to get their hearts to start beating. 'Greenies' are pep pills—dextroamphetamine sulfate. These players couldn't function without them." It is suggested by Bouton that more than half of major league ballplayers take amphetamines.

At an annual convention of the AMA in June 1970, Ohio

State's Doctor Murphy listed amphetamines as "number one" in terms of potential harm to athletes. Many times amphetamines are prescribed by doctors for various needs of the patient, but they can be highly toxic if consumed in quantity. The uppers are particularly hazardous to athletes because they artificially heighten the strain on different body systems. This energy strain coupled with the strain of athletic activity can become dangerous if not altogether fatal by causing cardiovascular collapse, cerebral hemorrhage, or brain lesions. Some of the less serious side effects of uppers are dizziness, nausea, headaches, agitation, and anxiety.

Among the most familiar amphetamines used by athletes are benzedrine, Dexedrine, Dexamyl, and methedrine ("speed").

Harold Connolly, a veteran of four U.S. Olympic teams, has said, "My experience tells me that an athlete will use *any* aid to improve his performance short of killing himself." It is a sad commentary indeed to think that the athletic attitude has been reduced to such a state.

Information and data about new drugs, fads, and gimmicks is constantly flowing into the sports world by way of professional publications, medical meetings, publications, and the athletic grapevine that joins all the locker rooms of the world.

The ugly cycle of drug abuse is summarized by a statement of an anonymous pro-football trainer, who says, "Some of the pros need almost a full week to get over getting pepped up for Sunday. Afterward they must either have tranquilizers or whiskey to bring them down. So they move through a cycle; pepped up, drunk, hung over, depressed, then pepped up again."

Barbiturates

Another class of drugs that are widely misused is the barbiturates. These are used to depress precompetition excitability and to encourage relaxation in events that require it by acting on the central nervous system. The effects vary from compound to compound, and some are associated with habit formation and dependence. Their use is common among professional football and hockey players as well as some amateurs. Their effect is especially attractive to this hard-driving group. Barbiturates dull the senses and depress the cardiac and respiratory centers, which are brought to a high pitch by the pressures and impact contact experienced by this type of athlete. These drugs also induce sleep in sufficient doses, thereby ensuring a good night's sleep the night before or after the game.

There are many barbiturates used by athletes including pentobarbitol (Nembutal), secobarbitol (Seconal), phenobarbitol (Luminal), and amobarbital (Amytal). The list keeps growing. The combination of uppers and downers, referred to as "greenies," has become popular with some athletes. Apparently the upper works to excite the pleasure and ego-support centers, while the downer decreases the usual attendant nervousness and shakiness of the upper. Research has validly proven that this combination does not increase efficiency and endurance; on the contrary, in most cases it serves to detract from athletic performance. However, the subjects feel their performance is improved because of the alteration of the ego view.

Hormonoids

Besides these mood-altering drugs there is a series of drugs called hormonoids. These drugs are synthetic reproductions of substances the body produces in varying amounts for body functioning.

1. Corticoid hormones and ACTH (adrenocorticotropic hormone) help to overcome extreme exhaustion. They also serve to reduce swelling and pain that may cause discomfort to the athlete. However, pain is an indicator of the body to warn against further activity or use of the particular area in pain. When pain is suppressed, the body is able to continue, thereby endangering its health. When used judiciously, in a moment of true need, these hormones are acceptable.

2. Thyroxin has a general stimulating effect on metabolism, resulting in increased combustion of glycogen, fat, and other metabolites, an increase in the oxygen requirement, and an increase in heat production. By its very nature this drug is harmful to the athlete. Nevertheless, it is generally used for weight reduction when a decrease is necessary for a particular event. These ends can and should be accomplished by more natural means, such as reduced intake of calories and carbohydrates and an increase in physical activity.

3. Insulin and adrenalin are two related drugs. Insulin enhances the uptake of glucose and potassium by the tissues, and adrenalin stimulates glucose metabolism in the cells. Pathological conditions may demand their use, but in healthy individuals the endocrine system handles their flow. When an athlete uses them to increase metabolism, it leads only to a disturbance of metabolic functioning.

4. The anabolic steroids are the only drugs used by athletes that have been found to have more than a temporary effect. It has been stated that 80 percent of weight lifters, shot-putters, discus throwers, and javelin throwers use these substances, which supposedly improve the assimilation of protein and thus encourage increased weight and muscle mass. They also enhance the formation of large glycogen stores.

Not long ago anabolic steroids were virtually unknown to American athletes; now they are talked about or used in every sport. The pioneer of these drugs in the American sports world was Dr. John Ziegler, an Olney, Maryland, physician. According to his own account, quoted in *Sports Illustrated*, Dr. Ziegler had heard that the Russian athletes were "bulking up" as a result of using hormones. Subsequently, Dr. Ziegler in cooperation with the CIBA Pharmaceutical Company began to administer these hormones to weight lifters at a Pennsylvania barbell club. The response was immediate and enthusiastic—too much so. Instead of taking the prescribed amount, the weight lifters figured two was better than one, so they consumed two or three times as many as directed. When Ziegler began to notice deleterious side effects such as prostate troubles and a few cases of atrophied testes, he discontinued the use of steroids.

The young male undergoes great changes in body weight and size and secondary sex characteristics at puberty. These changes are brought about by increased secretions of the androgenic hormones—the male sex hormones. There are five different androgen secretions from the adrenal gland, and others are derived from the testes. Testosterone is considered the androgen primarily responsible for male sex characteristics, because of the large quantity secreted by the body. Its major effect is to increase protein synthesis, which in turn accounts for the increased weight and size of the body. (This process by which food is built up into protoplasm or tissue is called anabolism.) Along with its anabolic effect on the body, testosterone has potent androgenic properties; if used therapeutically in women or children, it may lead to virilization. Consequently, biochemists have developed a variety of synthetic compounds to increase the anabolic properties of testosterone and decrease its androgenic effects. However, the efficacy of these anabolic steroids depends on adequate ingestion of protein and calories, along with physical activity.

Steroids seem to have three positive effects on athletes using them in proper doses.

1. Improvement of protein assimilation. Some gains in strength have been as high as 40 and 50 percent.

2. Promotion of calcium retention, which develops skeletal structure, thereby increasing height even in adults.

3. Aid to cell growth, which in turn increases body and muscle growth. Some athletes have gained 40 or 50 pounds in a few months.

Steroids have a therapeutic effect in the treatment of chronic debilitating illnesses, certain anemic conditions, male hormone deficiency, and osteoporosis (abnormal porousness of bones) and as an aid to the weakened elderly and those recovering from surgery. The problems in anabolic use occur when they are used by healthy young athletes.

Newsweek of December 29, 1969, reported that Brigitte Berendonk, a high-ranking 27-year-old West German discus thrower and shot-putter, said, "The hormone pill or shot is as much a part of modern competitive sport as the training program and the tricot sweat suit." According to Ms. Berendonk nearly all the world-class decathlon competitors, most discus throwers, shot-putters, and weight lifters, and half the runners and jumpers were using hormones. The article names American decathlon champions Bill Toomey and Russ Hodge, along with Swedish discus thrower Rickey Bruch, as taking hormone pills. "The practice is now so widespread that the younger groups who are just starting out have no choice if they want to stay on top," says Al Oerter, four-time Olympic discus champion.

A survey of 38 track and field athletes and weight lifters at UCLA discovered that fully half of them had taken or were taking one or more steroids. In many cases the amounts consumed were up to four times the prescribed therapeutic doses (normal recommended daily dose is 2 to 10 milligrams).

According to Dr. Tom Waddell, a practicing physician and decathlon performer at the Olympics in Mexico, over one-third of those on the U.S. track and field team were using anabolic steroids at the pre-Olympic training camp at South Lake Tahoe in 1968. The drug was taken orally by most, but some athletes were giving themselves injections with their own hypodermic syringes.

According to the *New York Times Magazine* (October 17, 1971) nearly all the Olympic hammer throwers, discus throwers, shot-putters, and other competitors in strength events were using steroids. Most of the top men in track and field have either publicly or privately admitted to having used steroids. According to *Sports Illustrated* this list includes Randy Matson, the 1968 Olympic Champion and world record holder in the shot put; Dallas Long, the 1964 Olympic shot put champion; and Hal Connolly, the 1956 Olympic champion in the hammer throw.

"Problems in a Turned-on World" (*Sports Illustrated*, June 23, 1969) claims that "based on reasonably good but unverifiable reports, some players on almost every NFL and AFL team have used anabolic steroids." In the same article Ken Ferguson, who went from Utah State University to Canadian pro football, claims that 90 percent of college linemen have used steroids. Ferguson was quoted as having said in 1968, "I'd say anybody who has graduated from college to pro football in the last four years has used them."

The use of steroids is not limited to pros and college athletes, but has of course precipitated to the high school athlete. It has been reported that many school basketball players have been using steroids in an attempt to gain height.

The athletes themselves are not solely to blame for the widespread use of these steroids. There are verified incidents where pro scouts have supplied the drug to college draftees and where college recruiters have given them to high school players. At the University of California it was the coaches and team physician who introduced steroids into the athletic program. According to reports the team physician at Berkeley prescribed steroids for any of the athletes who needed "beefing up." Steve McConnell, a former middle linebacker for the University of Southern California, said steroids were taken for granted as a normal part of training. This was the rule rather than the exception.

In some instances where steroids and other drugs have been forced on athletes, retaliation has occurred. The San Diego Chargers were accused of having freely dispensed both amphetamines and steroids by Paul Lowe, their former All-Pro running back. In testimony before a California legislative subcommittee inquiring into drug abuse in sport, Lowe claimed steroid pills were given to the players unknowingly at the dining table during training periods.

Dave Meggyesy, seven-year veteran linebacker for the

St. Louis Cardinals, wrote an autobiography called *Out of Their League.* He claimed that NFL trainers do more dealing in drugs than the average junkie. Meggyesy singled out the Cardinal trainer, Jack Rockwell, as having a "veritable drug-store" in his training room. After publication of the book Ken Gray, captain of the Cardinals and five-time veteran of the Pro Bowl, brought a $1.79-million law suit against the team, claiming that "potent, harmful, illegal and dangerous drugs" were dispensed to him without his consent.

According to a book published in 1969 (N.Y. Academy Press) called *Androgens and Anabolic Agents* by J. Vida there are no truly 100-percent anabolic steroids to date. All of them have some androgenic properties. The complete list of anabolic agents is over 600. Following is a list of a few commercial varieties, most of which are anabolic in nature.

Compound	Trade Name
ethylosestrenol	Maxibolin, or Orabolin
methandienone	Dianabol, or Danabol
methandriol	Stenediol
norethandrolone	Nilevar
nandrolone decanoate	deca-Durabolin, or Abolon
oxandrolone	Anavar
stanozolol	Winstrol, or Stromba

The predominance of anabolic steroids in training programs has prompted opposition to their use in athletics by the AMA's Committee on the Medical Aspects of Sports, the Committee on Sports Medicine of the American Academy of Sciences, the IAAF, the National Collegiate Athletic Association, the IOC, the FDA, and outstanding pharmaceutical organizations.

The decision to control the use of steroids was taken from the point of view of both athletic ethics and integrity and the still undetermined physiological hazards of prolonged use.

From all the data accumulated it appears that at this point there are both positive and negative reports. John P.

O'Shea and William Winkler of Oregon State University have done a great deal of research on the subject. In *Nutrition Report International* (December 1970) the extent and results of their experiment were published.

The purpose of the experiment was to evaluate the effects of an anabolic steroid (oxandrolone-"anavar") on (1) blood chemistry, (2) protein metabolism, and (3) performance (speed and strength) in competitive swimmers and weight lifters.

The volunteer subjects ranged from 18 to 25 years old. Eight of them were varsity swimmers, and three were competitive weight lifters. Five of the swimmers qualified for the National Collegiate Championships. Upon entering the study the swimmers had just completed three months of preseason conditioning that involved four hours of training per day. This training included weight lifting, calisthenics, and of course interval swim trainings.

The three weight lifters were of high caliber, too. One of them was an AAU champion in his body weight division. The lifters began the study after completing four months of preseason conditioning requiring an hour and a half of training a day, five days a week.

The duration of the study was eleven weeks. Along with 10 milligrams per day of oxandrolone for six weeks, a high-protein (86-percent) supplement was fed in the amount of half a gram per kilogram of body weight. Test results indicated no side effects such as edema or impaired liver function. Strength performance was significantly increased in the weight lifters, but there was no evidence that steroid treatment improved speed in the competitive swimmers. The report speculates that steroids may be administered in certain controlled situations, but it does not imply that anabolic steroids should be taken routinely by athletes. The conclusion claims that while there seem to be no serious side effects associated with short-term treatment (three to six weeks), long-term usage must be viewed with extreme caution.

A report by D. Freed in the *British Medical Journal* (3,

1972) of a double-blind study using Dianabol indicates results contrary to O'Shea's. Freed noted that low (10 milligrams per day) and high (25 milligrams per day) dosages of Dianabol in comparison with a placebo created problems with blood pressure and the prostate—and even caused acne in ten weight lifters. The conclusion was that it would not be wise to state that steroids at low levels have no adverse effects.

The most widely known research on steroid use was published in the *Journal of Applied Physiology* (20:1965) by Dr. William M. Fowler, Jr., formerly of UCLA Medical School. In a double-blind study Dr. Fowler found that the drug did not actually increase weight, but weight gains were due to fluid retention and did not necessarily result in strength increase. Dr. Fowler concluded that the increase in strength was in direct correlation to the amount of hard work and exercise in both drug users and nonusers.

These tests involved the administration of normal dosages. Some, probably most, athletes take much greater dosages. In those quantities—and even in normal quantities—anabolic steroids have been known to cause liver damage (chemical hepatitis), prostatic hypertrophy (enlarged prostate gland), testicular atrophy (shrunken testicles), and premature closure of the growing plates in the long bones in younger athletes. The younger the athlete taking the drug, the greater the probability his growth will be stunted. Steroids can also aggravate and stimulate the growth of any pre-existing cancers or hormone-sensitive tumors, and can result in decreased libido and infertility. In some cases gynecomastia (breast development) develops in male athletes.

Dr. Fowler said, "The use of androgens in athletics is unethical, and those using or administering them should be banned from further competition or professional activity."

In "Drugs and the Athlete" (*Reader's Digest*, September 1969) Dr. H. Kay Dooley, director of the Wood Memorial Clinic in Pomona, California, takes the opposite point of view:

I don't think it is possible for a weight man to compete internationally without using anabolic steroids. Many weight men on the Olympic team had to take steroids. Otherwise they would not have been in the running. If I know of something which may improve performance, a drug that is legal and which I don't believe involves any serious health risk, I see no reason not to make it available to an athlete when the need arises and under controlled administering procedures. I can't see an ethical difference between giving a drug to improve performance and wrapping an ankle or handing out a salt pill for the same purpose.

Perhaps the most serious and hazardous problem with male hormone drugs is their use by women. This has precipitated the "sex test"—a hormonal test accompanied by a gynecological examination—as a requirement for female athletes at the Olympic Games and other international sporting events. The first international competition to use this test was the 1966 European track and field championships. Five women, including the famous Press sisters of the Soviet Union, withdrew from competition rather than submit to the test. According to some reports their denial was not out of indignation but rather out of fear of not passing. It has been shown that long-term use of male hormones by women can cause the appearance of secondary male sex characteristics such as facial hair growth and baldness patterns. Their use by women is not advised by any authorities.

The drug controversy continues. The most tragic aspect of the problem is the fear that motivates drug use. What kind of misguided society pressures its athletes into thinking that their own self-destruction is worth the cost of winning? Athletes have become reduced to automatons, simply reacting to whatever chemical compounds are administered to them. Indeed, it is a rarity today to find any successful athlete who does not take drugs of some sort. Tom Ecker, a respected coach and author of six books on athletics, once said to a sportswriter, "I normally assume that the winner of a sports contest is one who has a better pharmacist than his opponent. In order to be in sports in the future it seems inconceivable that you could hold your own without drugs." This is indeed a sad commentary on the future of sports. The problem seems irretrievable. The most optimistic view holds some degree of hope in the young athletes who have not yet been ruined. The hope for the future lies in their outlook on life, self-image, and the respect given to parents and coaches. This respect can only be earned by a realistic and knowledgeable attitude toward drug misuse, a love of true sportsmanship, and an unequivocal desire for the healthy maturation of the young athlete.

Don Walter, Director of Physical Education and Athletics in the Upper St. Clair, Pennsylvania, School District has said:

> The athlete must learn that there is no short cut to success. The one chemical that can produce results is the perspiration which is the product of a sound program of physical conditioning and skill practice.
>
> Quite possibly the most important responsibility of the coach is to convince each athlete that he has a genuine interest in him that transcends the practice and playing field. The athlete must know that he has earned his coach's respect and willingness to help him with any problem that may confront him at any time during or after his athletic career. The coach is provided with a greater opportunity to develop a positive rapport with his students than any other member of the school staff. He sees the athlete in a variety of situations from the formality of the contest to the informality of the locker room. He sees the athlete exposed to emotional situations from the elation of success to the disappointment that comes from falling short. The athlete may well spend more time with the coach than with his own parents and

the coach is often the most respected and accessible friend to whom the young person can turn. The well-informed coach who makes himself available will be able to help.

8 MYTHS AND MISCONCEPTIONS ON NUTRITION AND ATHLETICS

There are some popular misconceptions among young athletes that need debunking. Following is a group of them, with the truth in each instance.

Misconception: Protein is the primary source of muscular energy.
Truth: Protein is not a major source of energy in a well-nourished person. Protein needs change with growth and the increased muscle mass that results from training.

Misconception: Steak is the best source of protein.
Truth: Fish and poultry are as valuable a source of protein as beef. So are pork, lamb, eggs, and dairy products.

Misconception: Eggs are the most important source of protein next to meat.
Truth: A properly cooked egg in any form is digested well and is a good source of protein—but it is no better than any other source of protein.

Misconception: Raw eggs are best.
Truth: Raw eggs can be most harmful. The danger is a chance of bacterial contamination with Salmonella, which causes food poisoning. In addition, raw eggs contain avi-

din, which destroys biotin. Avidin is neutralized in cooking. Cooked eggs are best nutritionally.

Misconception: A person should eat three or four eggs a day.

Truth: Current research seems to indicate that eggs should be curtailed to three or four per week by people with high cholesterol counts or a history of family heart disease. All others need not be so careful.

Misconception: Do not eat fats and fried foods—only salad dressings.

Truth: The body needs a certain amount of fat. A moderate amount of fried food is tolerated by a young body. In addition, fats are carriers of the fat-soluble vitamins (A, D, E, and K).

Misconception: Eat no sweets, and restrict bread and potatoes during training.

Truth: A certain amount of carbohydrates must be available to replace those burned up in training. It would be almost impossible to maintain a 3,000-calorie-a-day diet without some sugar and starches. Of course, these should be regulated.

Misconception: Stay away from irritating spices.

Truth: Pepper (white or black), chili peppers, cloves, and mustard seed should be limited by all. But such other spices as cinnamon, mace, thyme, sage, and paprika seem less irritating. This is a personal matter.

Misconception: For the pregame meal avoid bulky foods such as lettuce.

Truth: Lettuce actually contains less roughage (fiber content) than many other vegetables and fruits. (Check foods for fiber content.) It does not upset digestion, and contributes favorably to fecal bulk.

Misconception: It is best not to drink while eating.

Truth: It isn't harmful to drink while eating. Of course, it is not advisable to use water or other beverages to wash food down without chewing it. However, there are still enough digestive juices to handle even large gulps of food. Drinking can fill you up and kill your appetite, however.

Misconception: Don't drink ice water or cold drinks when eating.

Truth: Cold drinks should be drunk slowly. If taken in excess, they may interrupt normal peristalsis (digestive action).

Misconception: Don't drink water during practice. Just rinse out your mouth or suck on ice cubes.

Truth: Some water is necessary to combat dehydration. Water is lost in sweating and should be replaced hour by hour.

Misconception: Tea is the preferred drink prior to a game.

Truth: Both tea and coffee contain caffeine and are to be avoided before any game or meet. This consideration is often disregarded among coaches, and both are offered as a pregame liquid.

Misconception: Milk intake should be restricted.

Truth: Milk is an excellent source of protein and almost a perfect food. There is no scientific evidence that milk should be eliminated from the athlete's diet.

Misconception: Milk causes cotton mouth (dry mouth).

Truth: Saliva flow is influenced by dehydration and the emotional state of the athlete. No food or liquid causes it.

Misconception: Milk "cuts wind"—that is, it decreases performance.

Truth: Studies have shown there is no difference in training or performance whether or not milk is included in the diet.

Misconception: Milk causes sour stomach by curdling in the stomach.

Truth: On the contrary—milk may neutralize excess stomach

acid. The curdling that results when milk mixes with stomach acids is a necessary process of digestion.

Misconception: Honey is the best source of quick energy.
Truth: Honey is preferable to refined sugars but is not superior to other common sweets.

Misconception: Honey or other quick-energy foods before games or meets of short duration improve performance.
Truth: Energy needed for short-term performance is available in the body. Quick-energy food won't necessarily improve performance, but it will help the body replace energy used.

Misconception: Crash diets are OK on rare occasions.
Truth: These diets often hinder good health and performance. And the temptation to continue to use them over a long period of time adds to the danger of harmful metabolic effects.

Misconception: Vitamin supplementation is unimportant.
Truth: In light of current environmental stress some supplementation is necessary.

Misconception: Vitamin C doesn't help heal injuries.
Truth: Vitamin C helps the body to produce collagen, the cementing substance that holds body cells together. Collagen aids in forming strong scar tissue, which helps wounds heal, and it helps to resist infection. Since vitamin C passes through the body quickly, there is no chance of an overdose, and it can be taken freely.

9 CONCLUSION

In our attempt to accumulate information on nutrition and athletics we were shocked to discover that many supposedly well-informed athletes have little or no concern about diet. This seems quite alarming, much like a racing car driver placing little significance on the oils, tires, and engine components his car needs for maximum functioning.

ATHLETES WITH DIFFERENT PROGRAMS

The following random samples show how some Olympic athletes feel about diet and vitamin and mineral supplementation.

Sprinters

Kathy Hammond was a bronze medal winner for the women's 400-meter run in 1972. She takes . . . "no vitamin or mineral pills other than iron. However, I avoid greasy foods in the meal preceding the race."

Rod Milburn was the 1972 Olympic champion in the 110-meter high hurdles. "I eat no special foods. A lot of hard work is responsible for me winning the gold medal."

Eddie Hart and *Robert Taylor* were members of the XXth Olympic games gold-medal-winning 400-meter relay team. "We don't eat any special foods. We just get out and run."

John Smith, who was the world record-holder for the 440-yard run, said, "I take a multivitamin/mineral supplement and a protein supplement each day. I figure it's better to have too much than not enough."

Middle-Distance Runners

Dave Wottle was the world record-holder and 1972 Olympic champion in the 800-meter run. "I don't take anything artificial except Rolaids."

Jim Ryun, famous holder of the world record in the 1,500-meter run and the mile run, says "I eat no special foods and take no supplements."

Steve Prefontaine was the American record holder in the 3,000- and 5,000-meter runs. "I take a multivitamin each day and a breakfast drink that includes wheat germ oil. I don't know if it helps me, but it sure doesn't hurt."

Leonard Hilton was the national indoor champion in the three-mile run and stated that he is ". . . a strong believer in additional vitamins C, E, and B-complex tablets each day."

Field Events Competitors

Olga Connolly, former women's discus Olympic champion, says she takes no supplementation whatsoever.

Deanne Wilson, who was the American champion in the women's high jumps said, "I take 12 different vitamin and mineral pills every other day. I think they help me."

Ron Jourdan, who was the 1969 indoor national collegiate champion in the high jump, explained that he takes "a multivitamin and B-complex tablet, plus a vitamin E pill each day. I've been taking them for the last year and a half. I really don't think they help unless you aren't eating three square meals a day. However, they are especially important to me because I try to lose four or five pounds before an important competition. Besides, it's hard to really know what you're getting from most food you eat."

Al Feuerback, holder of the record for the indoor shot put, is an ardent believer in supplementation. "I take most all the supplements including a time-released vitamin/mineral powder, wheat germ oil, and protein pills."

George Frenn, who was the American record holder in the hammer throw, said, "I used to take vitamins by injection and eat many health foods, but not any more. I think they are all a bunch of hooey."

Dwight Stones, a 1972 bronze medal winner in the high jump, stated, "I take a multivitamin, plus additional C and E tablets each day. I think these help me guard against colds and infections."

Long-Distance Runners

Jack Bacheler, who was the 1969 AAU cross-country champion said, "I've gotten good results from eating a high-carbohydrate diet several days prior to my competition. Also, during my marathon running I will drink 64 ounces of uncarbonated Coke at intervals along the way. This seems to give me an additional kick."

Frank Shorter, Olympic marathon champion: "Three days prior to the marathon, I tried to load up on carbohydrates. I gained several pounds which I consider to be to my advantage as I have more energy. However, generally speaking, training is more important than nutrition."

Jeff Galloway was the American record holder for the 10 mile run and a ". . . firm believer in three balanced meals a day. Even if there were magic pills which would make me run faster, I'd rather know that I did it on my own."

Swimmers

Steve Genter, winner of a silver medal in the 1972 200-meter and 400-meter freestyle, said, "I try to stay away from foods with little nutritional value. I take no food supplements as I try to eat a balanced diet each day."

Doug Northway holds a bronze medal in the 1,500-meter freestyle and takes a ". . . multivitamin pill and several salt tablets daily during my training program."

Mark Spitz, most celebrated of the athletes of the Olympics in Munich for the XXth Games, had this to say: ". . . I don't take any supplements. But I have been eating yoghurt.

. . . Some of the swimmers are pill freaks, especially B6 and B12. I think it gives them just a mental lift or a type of placebo power."

Other Athletes

Phil Grippaldi of the U.S. weight lifting team and winner in the middle heavyweight class said, "I take seven individual vitamin pills at each meal and also a liver protein supplement. I've been taking them for so long that I don't want to stop taking them now. I can definitely feel a lag in my endurance when I quit taking wheat germ oil."

Tom Burleson of the U.S. basketball team said, "I eat lots of protein foods such as meat and milk. However, I take no pills or supplements."

Chris Taylor of the U.S. wrestling team: "I don't believe in supplements, just a lot of regular food."

Russ Knipp, U.S. weight lifting team: "I adhere to a high protein/low carbohydrate diet during training. In addition I take a multivitamin/mineral pill and wheat germ oil."

Ray Seales, Olympic winner of the light welterweight division boxing, said: "I don't eat any bread or starch. It makes me soft inside. I eat a lot of meat and green vegetables, and I also take a vitamin-mineral supplement."

As the reader can see, all these athletes have their own ideas on nutrition.

It seems incredible that many athletes who are looked up to as the paragons of physical health and culture take so little interest in diet and nutrition. If this disinterest and lack of knowledge is rampant among top athletes in the country, it is frightening to think of how little information has been disseminated to the average nonprofessional athlete.

SUMMARY

Athletes naturally look to their coaches for help and suggestions as they prepare for games or events. On every level the coach must serve as a counselor on dietary practice. He must warn his athletes about crash diets, unsound and sometimes highly dangerous fads concerning the relation of food and performance.

There is of course great stress on nutrition and diet in professional sports and even to some degree in collegiate sports. But by not stressing nutrition for children and teenagers coaches and parents are missing a great opportunity to help these youngsters. Proper nutritional guidance combined with a healthy attitude about sports can prepare girls and boys to lead longer, healthier, happier, and more rewarding lives.

A recent survey of high school coaches throughout the U.S. revealed a wide variety of nutritional and dietary suggestions and recommendations. Unfortunately, the majority of coaches in the survey based their recommendations on their own athletic experiences, and few consulted nutritionists, dieticians, or doctors. "Eat a balanced diet," seemed to be the advice. While this is sound, it is not enough.

Coaches have the responsibility to arm themselves with as much information on nutrition as possible.

They have an excellent opportunity to educate people about nutrition. Young athletes are highly motivated and therefore prime candidates for specific education on nutrition.

We feel that the relationship between sports and nutrition has not been investigated thoroughly and that all responsibly interested people should demand adequate investigation.

At all education levels the assistance of nutritionists and dieticians should be sought. Seminars and courses can be arranged for coaches, athletes, parents—indeed for all concerned with good health, for good health is a combination of proper nutrition with proper exercise.

As Senator William Proxmire of Wisconsin says, "Considering how little promotional effort is put into preventive health measures—promoting exercise, proper diet, and relaxation—our citizens have responded remarkably well.

"Although promotion of cigarettes, automobiles, television, and overeating must hit the average American a solid hundred times more frequently, not only in television and other media advertising but also in convenience and accessibility and especially in social acceptance, literally millions of Americans are battling against the tide, engaging in more exercise, following diets, and learning how to relax."

We must all contribute to winning that battle. The following organizations can assist the athlete in his search for nutritional information:

U.S. Dept. of Agriculture
Washington, D.C. 20402

American Association for Health, Physical Education and Recreation
1201 16th St. NW
Washington, D.C. 20036

American Dietetic Association
620 N. Michigan Ave
Chicago, Ill. 60611

American Heart Association
44 East 23rd Street
New York 10010

Nutrition Foundation
99 Park Ave.
New York 10016

National Dairy Council
111 N. Canal St.
Chicago Ill. 60606

Food and Nutrition Board—National Research Council
National Academy of Sciences
Washington, D.C.

World Health Organization
United Nations Plaza
New York 10017

APPENDIX

THE COMPOSITION OF FOODS

FOOD AND DESCRIPTION *(per 100 grams,* *edible portion)*	FOOD ENERGY	PROTEIN	FAT	CARBO- HYDRATE
Abalone:	*Calories*	*Grams*	*Grams*	*Grams*
Raw	98	18.7	0.5	3.4
Canned	80	16.0	.3	2.3
Almonds:				
Dried	598	18.6	54.2	19.5
Roasted and salted	627	18.6	57.7	19.5
Almond meal, partially defat- ted	408	39.5	18.3	28.9
Amaranth, raw	36	3.5	.5	6.5
Anchovy, pickled, with and without added oil, not heavily salted.	176	19.2	10.3	.3
Apples:				
Raw, commercial varieties:				
Freshly harvested and stored:				
Not pared	58	.2	.6	14.5
Pared	54	.2	.3	14.1
Freshly harvested:				
Not pared	56	.2	.6	14.1
Pared	53	.2	.3	13.9
Stored:				
Not pared	60	.2	.7	14.8
Pared	55	.2	.3	14.4
Dehydrated, sulfured:				
Uncooked	353	1.4	2.0	92.1
Cooked, with added sugar	76	.2	.3	19.6
Dried, sulfured:				
Uncooked	275	1.0	1.6	71.8

Source: USDA *Composition of Foods Handbook #8*

FOOD AND DESCRIPTION (per 100 grams, edible portion)	FOOD ENERGY Calories	PROTEIN Grams	FAT Grams	CARBO- HYDRATE Grams
Cooked:				
Without added sugar......	78	.3	.5	20.3
With added sugar............	112	.3	.4	29.2
Frozen, sliced, sweetened, not thawed	93	.2	.1	24.3
Apple brown betty	151	1.6	3.5	29.7
Apple butter	186	.4	.8	46.8
Apple juice, canned or bottled	47	.1	Trace	11.9
Applesauce, canned:				
Unsweetened or artificially sweetened	41	.2	.2	10.8
Sweetened	91	.2	.1	23.8
Apricots:				
Raw..............................	51	1.0	.2	12.8
Candied.....................	338	.6	.2	86.5
Apricot nectar, canned (approx. 40% fruit)	57	.3	.1	14.6
Artichokes, globe or French:				
Raw...	8-44	2.9	.2	10.6
Cooked, boiled, drained..........	8-44	2.8	.2	9.9
Asparagus:				
Raw spears...............................	26	2.5	.2	5.0
Cooked spears, boiled, drained	20	2.2	.2	3.6
Avocados, raw:				
All commercial varieties........	167	2.1	16.4	6.3
California, mainly Fuerte......	171	2.2	17.0	6.0
Florida	128	1.3	11.0	8.8
Bacon, cured:				
Raw, slab or sliced	665	8.4	69.3	1.0
Cooked, broiled or fried, drained	611	30.4	52.0	3.2
Canned	685	8.5	71.5	1.0
Bacon, Canadian:				
Unheated	216	20.0	14.4	.3
Cooked, broiled or fried, drained	277	27.6	17.5	.3
Bananas:				
Raw:				
Common	85	1.1	.2	22.2

FOOD AND DESCRIPTION *(per 100 grams, edible portion)*	FOOD ENERGY *Calories*	PROTEIN *Grams*	FAT *Grams*	CARBO-HYDRATE *Grams*
Red	90	1.2	.2	23.4
Dehydrated, or banana powder	340	4.4	.8	88.6
Barbecue sauce.........................	91	1.5	6.9	8.0
Barley, pearled:				
Light	349	8.2	1.0	78.8
Pot or Scotch	348	9.6	1.1	77.2
Barracuda, Pacific, raw	113	21.0	2.6	0
Bass, black sea:				
Raw...	93	19.2	1.2	0
Cooked, baked, stuffed	259	16.2	15.8	11.4
Bass, smallmouth and largemouth, raw	104	18.9	2.6	0
Bass, striped:				
Raw...	105	18.9	·2.7	0
Cooked, oven-fried..................	196	21.5	8.5	6.7
Bass, white, raw	98	18.0	2.3	0
Beans, common, mature seeds, dry:				
White:				
Raw......................................	340	22.3	1.6	61.3
Cooked	118	7.8	.6	21.2
Canned, solids and liquid:				
With pork and tomato sauce	122	6.1	2.6	19.0
With pork and sweet sauce	150	6.2	4.7	21.1
Without pork	120	6.3	.5	23.0
Red:				
Raw......................................	343	22.5	1.5	61.9
Cooked	118	7.8	.5	21.4
Canned, solids and liquid ..	90	5.7	.4	16.4
Pinto, calico, and red Mexican, raw	349	22.9	1.2	63.7
Other, including black, brown, and Bayo, raw	339	22.3	1.5	61.2
Beans, lima:				
Immature seeds:				
Raw......................................	123	8.4	.5	22.1
Cooked, boiled, drained	111	7.6	.5	19.8

FOOD AND DESCRIPTION (per 100 grams, edible portion)	FOOD ENERGY Calories	PROTEIN Grams	FAT Grams	CARBO-HYDRATE Grams
Canned:				
Regular pack:				
Solids and liquid..........	71	4.1	.3	13.4
Drained solids..............	96	5.4	.3	18.3
Drained liquid..............	20	1.3	Trace	3.9
Special dietary pack (low-sodium):				
Solids and liquid..........	70	4.4	.3	12.9
Drained solids..............	95	5.8	.3	17.7
Drained liquid..............	19	1.4	Trace	3.5
Frozen:				
Thick-seeded types, commonly called Fordhooks:				
Not thawed..................	102	6.2	0.1	19.5
Cooked boiled, drained	99	6.0	.1	19.1
Thin-seeded types, commonly called baby limas:				
Not thawed..................	122	7.6	.2	23.0
Cooked, boiled, drained	118	7.4	.2	22.3
Mature seeds, dry:				
Raw......................................	345	20.4	1.6	64.0
Cooked	138	8.2	.6	25.6
Bean flour, lima	343	21.5	1.4	63.0
Beans, mung:				
Mature seeds, dry, raw..........	340	24.2	1.3	60.3
Sprouted seeds:				
Uncooked	35	3.8	.2	6.6
Cooked, boiled, drained......	28	3.2	.2	5.2
Beans, snap:				
Green:				
Raw......................................	32	1.9	.2	7.1
Cooked, boiled, drained, cooked in—				
Small amount of water, short time	25	1.6	.2	5.4
Large amount of water, long time	25	1.6	.2	5.4

FOOD AND DESCRIPTION *(per 100 grams, edible portion)*	FOOD ENERGY *Calories*	PROTEIN *Grams*	FAT *Grams*	CARBO-HYDRATE *Grams*
Canned:				
Regular pack:				
Solids and liquid	18	1.0	.1	4.2
Beans and frankfurters, canned	144	7.6	7.1	12.6
Beaver, cooked, roasted	248	29.2	13.7	0
Beechnuts................................	568	19.4	50.0	20.3
Beef:				
Carcass:				
Total edible, including kidney and kidney fat, raw:				
Prime grade (54% lean, 46% fat)	428	13.6	41.	0
Choice grade (60% lean, 40% fat)	379	14.9	35.	0
Good grade (66% lean, 34% fat)	323	16.5	28.	0
Standard grade (73% lean, 27% fat)	266	18.0	21.	0
Commercial grade (64% lean, 36% fat)	347	15.8	31.	0
Utility grade (76% lean, 24% fat)	242	18.6	18.	0
Total edible, trimmed to retail level, raw:				
Choice grade (75% lean, 25% fat)	301	17.4	25.1	0
Good grade (78% lean, 22% fat)	263	18.5	20.4	0
Standard grade (82% lean, 18% fat)	225	19.4	15.8	0
Flank steak:				
Choice grade:				
Total edible:				
Raw (100% lean)	144	21.6	5.7	0
Cooked, braised (100% lean)	196	30.5	7.3	0
Good grade:				
Total edible:				

FOOD AND DESCRIPTION (per 100 grams, edible portion)	FOOD ENERGY Calories	PROTEIN Grams	FAT Grams	CARBO-HYDRATE Grams
Raw (100% lean)	139	21.8	5.1	0
Cooked, braised (100% lean)	191	30.8	6.6	0
Hindshank:				
Choice grade:				
Total edible:				
Raw (67% lean, 33% fat)	289	18.2	23.4	0
Cooked, simmered (66% lean, 34% fat)	361	25.1	28.1	0
Separable lean:				
Raw	134	21.7	4.6	0
Cooked, simmered	184	30.7	5.9	0
Separable fat:				
Raw	602	11.1	61.5	0
Good grade:				
Total edible:				
Raw (71% lean, 29% fat)	239	19.7	17.2	0
Cooked, simmered (70% lean, 30% fat)	307	27.2	21.1	0
Separable lean:				
Raw	126	21.8	3.7	0
Cooked, simmered	176	31.0	4.8	0
Separable fat:				
Raw	517	14.5	50.4	0
Loin or short loin:				
Porterhouse steak:				
Choice grade:				
Total edible:				
Raw (63% lean, 37% fat)	390	14.8	36.2	0
Cooked, broiled (57% lean, 43% fat)	465	19.7	42.2	0
T-bone steak:				
Choice grade:				
Total edible:				
Raw (62% lean, 38% fat)	397	14.7	37.1	0

FOOD AND DESCRIPTION *(per 100 grams, edible portion)*	FOOD ENERGY *Calories*	PROTEIN *Grams*	FAT *Grams*	CARBO-HYDRATE *Grams*
Cooked, broiled (56% lean, 44% fat)	473	19.5	43.2	0
Club steak:				
Choice grade:				
Total edible:				
Raw (64% lean, 36% fat)	380	15.5	34.8	0
Cooked, broiled (58% lean, 42% fat)	454	20.6	40.6	0
Round, entire (round and heel of round):				
Choice grade:				
Total edible:				
Raw (89% lean, 11% fat)	197	20.2	12.3	0
Cooked, broiled (81% lean, 19% fat)	261	28.6	15.4	0
Separable lean:				
Raw	135	21.6	4.7	0
Cooked, broiled	189	31.3	6.1	0
Separable fat:				
Raw	696	7.5	73.6	0
Rump:				
Choice grade:				
Total edible:				
Raw (75% lean, 25% fat)	303	17.4	25.3	0
Cooked, roasted (75% lean, 25% fat)	347	23.6	27.3	0
Separable lean:				
Raw	158	21.2	7.5	0
Cooked, roasted	208	29.1	9.3	0
Separable fat:				
Raw	726	6.2	77.6	0
Good grade:				
Total edible:				
Raw (76% lean, 24% fat)	271	18.3	21.4	0
Cooked, roasted (76% lean, 24% fat)	317	24.9	23.4	0

FOOD AND DESCRIPTION *(per 100 grams, edible portion)*	FOOD ENERGY *Calories*	PROTEIN *Grams*	FAT *Grams*	CARBO-HYDRATE *Grams*
Separable lean:				
Raw	141	21.6	5.4	0
Cooked, roasted	190	29.6	7.1	0
Separable fat:				
Raw	692	7.5	73.2	0
Hamburger (ground beef):				
Lean:				
Raw	179	20.7	10.0	0
Cooked...............................	219	27.4	11.3	0
Regular ground:				
Raw	268	17.9	21.2	0
Cooked...............................	286	24.2	20.3	0
Beef and vegetable stew:				
Cooked (home recipe, with lean beef chuck)	89	6.4	4.3	6.2
Canned	79	5.8	3.1	7.1
Beef, canned, roast beef........	224	25.	13.	0
Beef, corned, boneless:				
Uncooked, medium-fat	293	15.8	25.	0
Cooked, medium-fat................	372	22.9	30.4	0
Canned:				
Fat..	263	23.5	18.	0
Medium-fat	216	25.3	12.	0
Lean	185	26.4	8.	0
Canned corned-beef hash (with potato)	181	8.8	11.3	10.7
Beef, dried, chipped:				
Uncooked	203	34.3	6.3	0
Cooked, creamed	154	8.2	10.3	7.1
Beef potpie:				
Home-prepared, baked	246	10.1	14.5	18.8
Commercial, frozen, unheated	192	7.3	9.9	18.0
Beets, common, red:				
Raw..	43	1.6	.1	9.9
Cooked, boiled, drained..........	32	1.1	.1	7.2
Canned:				
Regular pack:				
Solids and liquid..............	34	0.9	0.1	7.9
Drained solids..................	37	1.0	.1	8.8
Drained liquid..................	26	.8	Trace	6.2

FOOD AND DESCRIPTION *(per 100 grams, edible portion)*	FOOD ENERGY *Calories*	PROTEIN *Grams*	FAT *Grams*	CARBO-HYDRATE *Grams*
Special dietary pack (low-sodium):				
Solids and liquid..............	32	.9	Trace	7.8
Drained solids..................	37	.9	.1	8.7
Drained liquid..................	25	.8	Trace	5.9
Beet greens, common:				
Raw...	24	2.2	.3	4.6
Cooked, boiled, drained..........	18	1.7	.2	3.3
Beverages, alcoholic and carbonated nonalcoholic:				
Alcoholic:				
Beer, alcohol 4.5% by volume (3.6% by weight)	42	.3	0	3.8
Gin, rum, vodka, whisky:				
80-proof (33.4% alcohol by weight)	231	—	—	Trace
86-proof (36.0% alcohol by weight)	249	—	—	Trace
90-proof (37.9% alcohol by weight)	263	—	—	Trace
94-proof (39.7% alcohol by weight)	275	—	—	Trace
100-proof (42.5% alcohol by weight)	295	—	—	Trace
Wines:				
Dessert, alcohol 18.8% by volume (15.3% by weight).	137	.1	0	7.7
Table, alcohol 12.2% by volume (9.9% by weight).	85	.1	0	4.2
Carbonated, nonalcoholic:				
Carbonated waters:				
Sweetened (quinine sodas)	31	(0)	(0)	8.
Unsweetened (club sodas)	0	(0)	(0)	0.
Cola type...............................	39	(0)	(0)	10.
Cream sodas........................	43	(0)	(0)	11.

FOOD AND DESCRIPTION (per 100 grams, edible portion)	FOOD ENERGY Calories	PROTEIN Grams	FAT Grams	CARBO-HYDRATE Grams
Fruit-flavored sodas (citrus, cherry, grape, strawberry, Tom Collins mixer, other) (10%–13% sugar).	46	(0)	(0)	12.
Ginger ale, pale dry and golden	31	(0)	(0)	8.
Root beer	41	(0)	(0)	10.5
Special dietary drinks with artificial sweetener (less than 1 calorie per ounce).	—	(0)	(0)	—
Biscuits, baking powder, baked from home recipe, made with—				
Enriched flour	369	7.4	17.0	45.8
Unenriched flour	369	7.4	17.0	45.8
Self-rising flour, enriched	372	7.1	17.4	46.0
Biscuit dough, commercial, with enriched flour:				
Chilled in cans	277	7.3	6.4	46.4
Frozen.......................................	327	5.7	11.9	48.9
Biscuit mix, with enriched flour, and biscuits baked from mix:				
Mix, dry form	424	7.7	12.6	68.7
Biscuits, made with milk....	325	7.1	9.3	52.3
Blackberries, including dewberries, boysenberries and youngberries, raw.	58	1.2	.9	12.9
Blackberries, canned, solids and liquid:				
Water pack, with or without artificial sweetener	40	.8	.6	9.0
Juice pack.................................	54	.8	.8	12.1
Sirup pack:				
Light	72	.8	.6	17.3
Heavy	91	.8	.6	22.2
Extra heavy	110	.8	.6	27.1
Blackberry juice, canned, unsweetened	37	.3	.6	7.8

FOOD AND DESCRIPTION *(per 100 grams, edible portion)*	FOOD ENERGY *Calories*	PROTEIN *Grams*	FAT *Grams*	CARBO-HYDRATE *Grams*
Blueberries:				
Raw..	62	.7	.5	15.3
Canned, solids and liquid:				
Water pack, with or without artificial sweetener	39	.5	.2	9.8
Sirup pack, extra heavy	101	.4	.2	26.0
Frozen, not thawed:				
Unsweetened	55	.7	.5	13.6
Sweetened.............................	105	.6	.3	26.5
Bluefish:				
Raw..	117	20.5	3.3	0
Cooked:				
Baked or broiled	159	26.2	5.2	0
Fried	205	22.7	9.8	4.7
Bonito, including Atlantic, Pacific, and striped; raw	168	24.0	7.3	0
Boston brown bread	211	5.5	1.3	45.6
Bouillon cubes or powder	120	20.	3.	5.
Boysenberries:				
Canned, water pack, solids and liquid, with or without artificial sweetener.	36	.7	.1	9.1
Frozen, not thawed:				
Unsweetened	48	1.2	.3	11.4
Sweetened.............................	96	.8	.3	24.4
Brains, all kinds (beef, calf, hog, sheep), raw	125	10.4	8.6	.8
Bran:				
Added sugar and malt extract	240	12.6	3.0	74.3
Added sugar and defatted wheat germ	238	10.8	1.8	78.8
Bran flakes (40% bran), added thiamine	303	10.2	1.8	80.6
Bran flakes with raisins, added thiamine	287	8.3	1.4	79.3
Brazilnuts..................................	654	14.3	66.9	10.9
Breads:				
Cracked-wheat	263	8.7	2.2	52.1
Toasted	313	10.4	2.6	62.0
French or vienna:				
Enriched	290	9.1	3.0	55.4

FOOD AND DESCRIPTION (per 100 grams, edible portion)	FOOD ENERGY Calories	PROTEIN Grams	FAT Grams	CARBO-HYDRATE Grams
Toasted	338	10.6	2.5	64.4
Unenriched	290	9.1	3.0	55.4
Toasted	338	10.6	3.5	64.4
Italian:				
Enriched	276	9.1	.8	56.4
Unenriched	276	9.1	.8	56.4
Raisin	262	6.6	2.8	53.6
Toasted	316	8.0	3.4	64.6
Rye:				
American (1/3 rye, 2/3 clear flour)	243	9.1	1.1	52.1
Toasted	282	10.6	1.3	60.5
Pumpernickel	246	9.1	1.2	53.1
Salt-rising	267	7.9	2.4	52.2
Toasted	297	8.8	2.7	58.0
White:				
Enriched, made with—				
1%–2% nonfat dry milk	269	8.7	3.2	50.4
Toasted	314	10.1	3.7	58.7
3%–4% nonfat dry milk	270	8.7	3.2	50.5
Toasted	314	10.1	3.7	58.8
5%–6% nonfat dry milk	275	9.0	3.8	50.2
Toasted	320	10.5	4.4	58.4
Unenriched, made with—				
1%–2% nonfat dry milk	269	8.7	3.2	50.4
Toasted	314	10.1	3.7	58.7
3%–4% nonfat dry milk	270	8.7	3.2	50.5
Toasted	314	10.1	3.7	58.8
5%–6% nonfat dry milk	275	9.0	3.8	50.2
Toasted	320	10.5	4.4	58.4
Whole-wheat, made with—				
2% nonfat dry milk	243	10.5	3.0	47.7
Toasted	289	12.5	3.6	56.7
Water	241	9.1	2.6	49.3
Toasted	287	10.8	3.1	58.7
Breadcrumbs, dry, grated	392	12.6	4.6	73.4
Bread pudding with raisins	187	5.6	6.1	28.4
Bread stuffing mix and stuffings prepared from mix:				
Mix, dry form	371	12.9	3.8	72.4

FOOD AND DESCRIPTION *(per 100 grams, edible portion)*	FOOD ENERGY *Calories*	PROTEIN *Grams*	FAT *Grams*	CARBO-HYDRATE *Grams*
Stuffing:				
Dry, crumbly: prepared with water, table fat	358	6.5	21.8	35.6
Moist: prepared with water, egg, table fat	208	4.4	12.8	19.7
Breadfruit, raw	103	1.7	.3	26.2
Broadbeans, raw:				
Immature seeds	105	8.4	.4	17.8
Mature seeds, dry	338	25.1	1.7	58.2
Broccoli:				
Raw spears..............................	32	3.6	.3	5.9
Cooked spears, boiled, drained	26	3.1	.3	4.5
Frozen:				
Chopped:				
Not thawed.......................	29	3.2	.3	5.2
Cooked, boiled, drained ..	26	2.9	.3	4.6
Spears:				
Not thawed.......................	28	3.3	.2	5.1
Cooked, boiled, drained ..	26	3.1	.2	4.7
Brussels sprouts:				
Raw......................................	45	4.9	.4	8.3
Cooked, boiled, drained..........	36	4.2	.4	6.4
Frozen:				
Not thawed...........................	36	3.3	.2	7.3
Cooked, boiled, drained	33	3.2	.2	6.5
Buckwheat:				
Whole-grain	335	11.7	2.4	72.9
Butter	716	.6	81.	.4
Butter oil or dehydrated butter	876	.3	99.5	0
Butterfish, raw:				
From northern waters	169	18.1	10.2	0
From gulf waters	95	16.2	2.9	0
Buttermilk:				
Fluid, cultured (made from skim milk)	36	3.6	.1	5.1
Dried......................................	387	34.3	5.3	50.0
Butternuts	629	23.7	61.2	8.4

FOOD AND DESCRIPTION (per 100 grams, edible portion)	FOOD ENERGY Calories	PROTEIN Grams	FAT Grams	CARBO-HYDRATE Grams
Cabbage:				
Common varieties (Danish, domestic, and pointed types):				
Raw..................................	24	1.3	.2	5.4
Cooked, boiled until tender, drained:				
Shredded, cooked in small amount of water	20	1.1	.2	4.3
Wedges, cooked in large amount of water	18	1.0	.2	4.0
Dehydrated...........................	308	12.4	1.7	73.7
Red, raw..................................	31	2.0	.2	6.9
Savoy, raw	24	2.4	.2	4.6
Cabbage, Chinese (also called celery cabbage or petsai), compact heading type, raw.	14	1.2	.1	3.0
Cabbage, spoon (also called white mustard cabbage or pakchoy), nonheading green leaf type:				
Raw..	16	1.6	.2	2.9
Cooked, boiled, drained..........	14	1.4	.2	2.4
Cakes:				
Baked from home recipes:				
Angelfood.............................	269	7.1	.2	60.2
Boston cream pie	302	5.0	9.4	49.9
Caramel:				
Without icing	385	4.5	17.3	53.7
With caramel icing..........	379	3.7	14.8	59.1
Chocolate (devil's food):				
Without icing	366	4.8	17.2	52.0
With chocolate icing	369	4.5	16.4	55.8
With uncooked white icing	369	3.8	14.6	59.2
Cottage pudding, made with enriched flour:				
Without sauce...................	344	6.4	11.3	54.3

FOOD AND DESCRIPTION *(per 100 grams, edible portion)*	FOOD ENERGY Calories	PROTEIN Grams	FAT Grams	CARBO- HYDRATE Grams
With chocolate sauce	318	5.3	8.8	56.7
With fruit sauce (straw-berry)	292	5.1	8.8	48.4
Fruitcake, made with en-riched flour:				
Dark	379	4.8	15.3	59.7
Light	389	6.0	16.5	57.4
Gingerbread, made with en-riched flour	317	3.8	10.7	52.0
Plain cake or cupcake:				
Without icing	364	4.5	13.9	55.9
With chocolate icing	368	4.2	13.9	59.4
With boiled white icing ..	352	3.8	10.5	61.8
With uncooked white ic-ing	367	3.4	11.8	63.3
Pound:				
Old-fashioned (equal weights flour, sugar, table fat, eggs).	473	5.7	29.5	47.0
Modified............................	411	6.4	18.7	54.7
Sponge	297	7.6	5.7	54.1
White:				
Without icing	375	4.6	16.0	54.0
With coconut icing	371	3.7	13.3	60.7
With uncooked white ic-ing	375	3.3	12.9	62.9
Yellow:				
Without icing	363	4.5	12.7	58.2
With caramel icing..........	362	4.0	11.7	61.3
With chocolate icing	365	4.2	13.0	60.4
Frozen, commercial, devil's food:				
With chocolate icing	380	4.3	17.6	55.6
With whipped-cream filling, chocolate icing	371	3.5	21.9	43.8
Cake mixes and cakes baked from mixes:				
Angelfood:				
Mix, dry form......................	385	8.4	0.2	88.5

FOOD AND DESCRIPTION (per 100 grams, edible portion)	FOOD ENERGY Calories	PROTEIN Grams	FAT Grams	CARBO- HYDRATE Grams
Cake, made with water, flavorings	259	5.7	.2	59.4
Chocolate malt:				
Mix, dry form......................	412	4.0	10.7	79.0
Cake, made with eggs, water, uncooked white icing.	346	3.4	8.7	66.6
Coffeecake, with enriched flour:				
Mix, dry form......................	431	5.9	11.0	77.2
Cake, made with egg, milk	322	6.3	9.6	52.4
Cupcake:				
Mix, dry form......................	438	3.7	13.6	75.8
Cake, made with eggs, milk, without icing	350	4.9	12.0	55.8
Cake, made with eggs, milk, chocolate icing	358	4.5	12.6	59.2
Devil's food:				
Mix, dry form......................	406	4.8	11.7	77.0
Cake, made with eggs, water, chocolate ic- ing	339	4.4	12.3	58.3
Gingerbread:				
Mix, dry form......................	425	5.4	10.4	78.2
Cake, made with water ..	276	3.1	6.8	51.1
Honey spice:				
Mix, dry form......................	443	4.3	14.0	76.3
Cake, made with eggs, water, caramel icing	352	4.1	10.8	60.9
Marble:				
Mix, dry form......................	425	4.9	13.5	75.6
Cake, made with eggs, water, boiled white icing	331	4.4	8.7	62.0
White:				
Mix, dry form......................	434	4.1	11.9	78.4
Cake, made with egg whites, water, choco- late icing.	351	3.9	10.7	62.8

FOOD AND DESCRIPTION (per 100 grams, edible portion)	FOOD ENERGY Calories	PROTEIN Grams	FAT Grams	CARBO- HYDRATE Grams
Yellow:				
Mix, dry form......................	438	4.0	12.9	77.6
Cake, made with eggs, water, chocolate icing	337	4.1	11.3	57.6
Cake icings:				
Caramel	360	1.3	6.7	76.5
Chocolate	376	3.2	13.9	67.4
Coconut...................................	364	1.9	7.7	74.9
White:				
Uncooked	376	.5	6.6	81.6
Boiled	316	1.4	0	80.3
Cake icing mixes and icings made from mixes:				
Chocolate fudge:				
Mix, dry form......................	409	2.5	9.8	86.4
Icing, made with water, table fat	378	2.2	14.4	67.0
Creamy fudge (contains nonfat dry milk):				
Mix, dry form......................	386	3.2	7.4	85.1
Icing:				
Made with water	339	2.8	6.5	74.6
Made with water, table fat	383	2.6	15.2	65.9
Candy:				
Butterscotch............................	397	Trace	3.4	94.8
Caramels:				
Plain or chocolate	399	4.0	10.2	76.6
Plain or chocolate, with nuts	428	4.5	16.3	70.5
Chocolate-flavored roll........	396	2.2	8.2	82.7
Chocolate:				
Bittersweet............................	477	7.9	39.7	46.8
Semisweet.............................	507	4.2	35.7	57.0
Sweet.....................................	528	4.4	35.1	57.9
Chocolate, milk:				
Plain	520	7.7	32.3	56.9
With almonds	532	9.3	35.6	51.3
With peanuts	543	14.1	38.1	44.6

FOOD AND DESCRIPTION (per 100 grams, edible portion)	FOOD ENERGY Calories	PROTEIN Grams	FAT Grams	CARBO-HYDRATE Grams
Chocolate-coated:				
Almonds	569	12.3	43.7	39.6
Chocolate fudge	430	3.8	16.0	73.1
Chocolate fudge, with nuts	452	4.9	20.8	67.3
Coconut center	438	2.8	17.6	72.0
Fondant.................................	410	1.7	10.5	81.0
Fudge, caramel, and peanuts	433	7.7	18.1	64.1
Fudge, peanuts, and caramel	459	9.4	23.1	58.7
Honeycombed hard candy, with peanut butter	463	6.6	19.5	70.6
Nougat and caramel	416	4.0	13.9	72.8
Peanuts.................................	561	16.4	41.3	39.1
Raisins	425	5.4	17.1	70.5
Vanilla creams	435	3.8	17.1	70.3
Fondant	364	.1	2.0	89.6
Fudge:				
Chocolate	400	2.7	12.2	75.0
Chocolate, with nuts	426	3.9	17.4	69.0
Vanilla.................................	398	3.0	11.1	74.8
Vanilla, with nuts	424	4.2	16.4	68.8
Gum drops, starch jelly pieces	347	.1	.7	87.4
Hard	386	0	1.1	97.2
Jelly beans	367	Trace	.5	93.1
Marshmallows	319	2.0	Trace	80.4
Peanut bars	515	17.5	32.2	47.2
Peanut brittle (no added salt or soda)	421	5.7	10.4	81.0
Sugar-coated:				
Almonds	456	7.8	18.6	70.2
Chocolate discs.....................	466	5.2	19.7	72.7
Carrots:				
Raw...	42	1.1	.2	9.7
Cooked, boiled, drained..........	31	.9	.2	7.1
Canned:				
Regular pack:				
Solids and liquid..............	28	.6	.2	6.5
Drained solids..................	30	.8	.3	6.7
Drained liquid.................	22	.4	0	5.5

FOOD AND DESCRIPTION (per 100 grams, edible portion)	FOOD ENERGY Calories	PROTEIN Grams	FAT Grams	CARBO-HYDRATE Grams
Special dietary pack (low-sodium):				
Solids and liquid..............	22	.7	.1	5.0
Drained solids.................	25	.8	.1	5.6
Drained liquid.................	16	.4	0	4.0
Dehydrated..............................	341	6.6	1.3	81.1
Cashew nuts	561	17.2	45.7	29.3
Catfish, freshwater, raw..........	103	17.6	3.1	0
Cauliflower:				
Raw...	27	2.7	.2	5.2
Cooked, boiled, drained..........	22	2.3	.2	4.1
Frozen:				
Not thawed..........................	22	2.0	.2	4.3
Cooked, boiled, drained......	18	1.9	.2	3.3
Caviar, sturgeon:				
Granular...................................	262	26.9	15.0	3.3
Pressed....................................	316	34.4	16.7	4.9
Celeriac, root, raw	40	1.8	.3	8.5
Celery, all, including green and yellow varieties:				
Raw...	17	.9	.1	3.9
Cooked, boiled, drained..........	14	.8	.1	3.1
Chard, Swiss:				
Raw...	25	2.4	0.3	4.6
Cooked, boiled, drained..........	18	1.8	.2	3.3
Charlotte russe, with ladyfingers, whipped-cream filling.	286	5.9	14.6	33.5
Chayote, raw	28	.6	.1	7.1
Cheeses, natural and processed; cheese foods; cheese spreads:				
Natural cheeses:				
Blue or Roquefort type......	368	21.5	30.5	2.0
Brick	370	22.2	30.5	1.9
Camembert (domestic)........	299	17.5	24.7	1.8
Cheddar (domestic type, commonly called American).	398	25.0	32.2	2.1
Cottage (large or small curd):				

FOOD AND DESCRIPTION (per 100 grams, edible portion)	FOOD ENERGY Calories	PROTEIN Grams	FAT Grams	CARBO-HYDRATE Grams
Creamed	106	13.6	4.2	2.9
Uncreamed	86	17.0	.3	2.7
Cream	374	8.0	37.7	2.1
Limburger	345	21.2	28.0	2.2
Parmesan	393	36.0	26.0	2.9
Swiss (domestic)	370	27.5	28.0	1.7
Pasteurized process cheese:				
American	370	23.2	30.0	1.9
Pimiento (American)	371	23.0	30.2	1.8
Swiss	355	26.4	26.9	1.6
Pasteurized process cheese food, American	323	19.8	24.0	7.1
Pasteurized process cheese spread, American	288	16.0	21.4	8.2
Cheese fondue, from home recipe	265	14.8	18.3	10.0
Cheese souffle, from home recipe	218	9.9	17.1	6.2
Cheese straws	453	11.2	29.9	34.5
Cherimoya, raw	94	1.3	.4	24.0
Cherries:				
Raw:				
Sour, red	58	1.2	.3	14.3
Sweet	70	1.3	.3	17.4
Candied	339	.5	.2	86.7
Canned:				
Sour, red, solids and liquid:				
Water pack	43	.8	.2	10.7
Sirup pack:				
Light	74	.8	.2	18.7
Heavy	89	.8	.2	22.7
Extra heavy	112	.8	.2	28.6
Sweet, solids and liquid:				
Water pack, with or without artificial sweetener	48	.9	.2	11.9
Sirup pack:				
Light	65	.9	.2	16.5
Heavy	81	.9	.2	20.5
Extra heavy	100	.8	.2	25.6

FOOD AND DESCRIPTION *(per 100 grams, edible portion)*	FOOD ENERGY Calories	PROTEIN Grams	FAT Grams	CARBO-HYDRATE Grams
Frozen, not thawed:				
Sour, red:				
Unsweetened	55	1.0	.4	13.4
Sweetened	112	1.0	.4	27.8
Cherries, maraschino, bottled, solids and liquid	116	.2	.2	29.4
Chervil, raw	57	3.4	.9	11.5
Chestnuts:				
Fresh..	194	2.9	1.5	42.1
Dried.......................................	377	6.7	4.1	78.6
Chicken:				
All classes:				
Light meat without skin:				
Raw	117	23.4	1.9	0
Cooked, roasted	166	31.6	3.4	0
Dark meat without skin:				
Raw	130	20.6	4.7	0
Cooked, roasted	176	28.0	6.3	0
Chicken, canned, meat only, boned	198	21.7	11.7	0
Chicken a la king, cooked, from home recipe	191	11.2	14.0	5.0
Chicken fricassee, cooked, from home recipe	161	15.3	9.3	3.2
Chicken potpie:				
Home-prepared, baked	235	10.1	13.5	18.3
Commercial, frozen, unheated	219	6.7	11.5	22.2
Chicken and noodles, cooked, from home recipe	153	9.3	7.7	10.7
Chickpeas or garbanzos, mature seeds, dry, raw	360	20.5	4.8	61.0
Chicory, Witloof (also called French or Belgian endive), bleached head (forced), raw.	15	1.0	.1	3.2
Chicory greens, raw	20	1.8	.3	3.8
Chili con carne, canned:				
With beans..............................	133	7.5	6.1	12.2
Without beans	200	10.3	14.8	5.8
Chives, raw	28	1.8	.3	5.8

FOOD AND DESCRIPTION (per 100 grams, edible portion)	FOOD ENERGY Calories	PROTEIN Grams	FAT Grams	CARBO-HYDRATE Grams
Chocolate:				
Bitter or baking......................	505	10.7	53.0	28.9
Chocolate sirup:				
Thin type	245	2.3	2.0	62.7
Fudge type...............................	330	5.1	13.7	54.0
Chop suey, with meat:				
Cooked, from home recipe	120	10.4	6.8	5.1
Canned	62	4.4	3.2	4.2
Chow mein, chicken (without noodles):				
Cooked, from home recipe	102	12.4	4.0	4.0
Canned	38	2.6	.1	7.1
Chub, raw...................................	145	15.3	8.8	0
Citron, candied...........................	314	.2	.3	80.2
Clams, raw:				
Soft:				
Meat and liquid	54	8.6	1.0	2.0
Meat only	82	14.0	1.9	1.3
Hard or round:				
Meat and liquid	49	6.5	.4	4.2
Meat only	80	11.1	.9	5.9
Hard, soft, and unspecified:				
Meat and liquid	53	8.1	.9	2.5
Meat only	76	12.6	1.6	2.0
Clams, canned, including hard, soft, razor, and un-specified:				
Solids and liquid	52	7.9	.7	2.8
Drained solids	98	15.8	2.5	1.9
Liquor, bouillon, or nectar	19	2.3	.1	2.1
Clam fritters	311	11.4	15.0	30.9
Cocoa and chocolate-fla-vored beverage powders:				
Cocoa powder with nonfat dry milk	359	18.6	2.9	70.8
Cocoa powder without milk ..	347	4.0	2.0	89.4
Mix for hot chocolate	392	9.4	10.6	73.9
Cocoa, dry powder:				
High-fat or breakfast:				
Plain	299	16.8	23.7	48.3

FOOD AND DESCRIPTION (per 100 grams, edible portion)	FOOD ENERGY Calories	PROTEIN Grams	FAT Grams	CARBO-HYDRATE Grams
Processed with alkali..........	295	16.8	23.7	45.4
Medium-fat:				
High-medium fat:				
Plain	265	17.3	19.0	51.5
Processed with alkali......	261	17.3	19.0	48.5
Low-medium fat:				
Plain	220	19.2	12.7	53.8
Processed with alkali......	215	19.2	12.7	50.2
Low-fat.....................................	187	20.2	7.9	58.0
Coconut cream (liquid expressed from grated coconut meat).	334	4.4	32.2	8.3
Coconut meat:				
Fresh..	346	3.5	35.3	9.4
Dried:				
Unsweetened	662	7.2	64.9	23.0
Sweetened, shredded..........	548	3.6	39.1	53.2
Coconut milk (liquid expressed from mixture of grated coconut meat and water).	252	3.2	24.9	5.2
Coconut water (liquid from coconuts)	22	.3	.2	4.7
Cod:				
Raw...	78	17.6	.3	0
Cooked, broiled	170	28.5	5.3	0
Canned	85	19.2	.3	0
Dehydrated, lightly salted	375	81.8	2.8	0
Dried, salted............................	130	29.0	.7	0
Coffee, instant, water-soluble solids:				
Dry powder	129	Trace	Trace	(35.)
Beverage..............................	1	Trace	Trace	Trace
Coleslaw, made with—				
French dressing (homemade)	129	1.1	12.3	5.1
French dressing (commercial)	95	1.2	7.3	7.6
Mayonnaise	144	1.3	14.0	4.8
Salad dressing (mayonnaise type)	99	1.2	7.9	7.1

FOOD AND DESCRIPTION (per 100 grams, edible portion)	FOOD ENERGY Calories	PROTEIN Grams	FAT Grams	CARBO-HYDRATE Grams
Cookies:				
Assorted, packaged, commercial	480	5.1	20.2	71.0
Brownies with nuts:				
Baked from home recipe, enriched flour	485	6.5	31.3	50.9
Frozen, with chocolate icing, commercial	419	4.9	20.6	60.7
Butter, thin, rich	457	6.1	16.9	70.9
Chocolate	445	7.1	15.7	71.5
Chocolate chip:				
Baked from home recipe, enriched flour	516	5.4	30.1	60.1
Commercial type	471	5.4	21.0	69.7
Coconut bars	494	6.2	24.5	63.9
Fig bars	358	3.9	5.6	75.4
Gingersnaps	420	5.5	8.9	79.8
Ladyfingers	360	7.8	7.8	64.5
Macaroons	475	5.3	23.2	66.1
Marshmallow	409	4.0	13.2	72.3
Molasses	422	6.4	10.6	76.0
Oatmeal with raisins	451	6.2	15.4	73.5
Peanut.....................................	473	10.0	19.1	67.0
Raisin	379	4.4	5.3	80.8
Sandwich type	495	4.8	22.5	69.3
Shortbread	498	7.2	23.1	65.1
Sugar, soft, thick, with enriched flour, home recipe	444	6.0	16.8	68.0
Sugar wafers	485	4.9	19.4	73.4
Vanilla wafers	462	5.4	16.1	74.4
Corn, field, whole-grain, raw ..	348	8.9	3.9	72.2
Corn, sweet:				
Raw, white and yellow	96	3.5	1.0	22.1
Cooked, boiled, drained, white and yellow:				
Kernels, cut off cob before cooking	83	3.2	1.0	18.8
Kernels, cooked on cob	91	3.3	1.0	21.0
Canned:				
Regular pack:				

FOOD AND DESCRIPTION (per 100 grams, edible portion)	FOOD ENERGY Calories	PROTEIN Grams	FAT Grams	CARBO-HYDRATE Grams
Cream style, white and yellow:				
Solids and liquid	82	2.1	.6	20.0
Whole kernel:				
Vacuum pack, yellow:				
Solids and liquid	83	2.5	.5	20.5
Wet pack, white and yellow:				
Solids and liquid	66	1.9	.6	15.7
Drained solids	84	2.6	.8	19.8
Drained liquid	26	.5	Trace	6.9
Corn products used mainly as ready-to-eat breakfast cereals:				
Corn flakes:				
Added nutrients	386	7.9	.4	85.3
Added nutrients, sugar-covered	386	4.4	.2	91.3
Corn, puffed:				
Added nutrients	399	8.1	4.2	80.8
Presweetened:				
Added nutrients	379	4.0	.2	89.8
Cocoa-flavored, added nutrients	390	6.2	2.2	86.7
Fruit-flavored, added nutrients	395	5.6	2.7	87.4
Corn, shredded, added nutrients	389	7.0	.4	86.9
Corn, rice, and wheat flakes, mixed, added nutrients	389	7.4	.7	86.1
Corn, flaked, with protein concentrate (casein) and other added nutrients.	378	23.0	1.6	67.0
Corn pudding	104	4.0	4.7	13.0
Cornbread, baked from home recipes:				
Cornbread, southern style, made with—				
Whole-ground cornmeal	207	7.4	7.2	29.1

FOOD AND DESCRIPTION (per 100 grams, edible portion)	FOOD ENERGY Calories	PROTEIN Grams	FAT Grams	CARBO-HYDRATE Grams
Degermed cornmeal, enriched	224	7.1	6.0	34.7
Johnnycake (northern style cornbread), made with enriched, yellow degermed cornmeal.	267	8.7	5.2	45.5
Corn pone, made with white, whole-ground cornmeal	204	4.5	5.3	36.2
Spoonbread, made with white whole-ground cornmeal.	195	6.7	11.4	16.9
Cowpeas, including blackeye peas:				
Immature seeds:				
Raw	127	9.0	.8	21.8
Cooked, boiled, drained	108	8.1	.8	18.1
Canned, solids and liquid ..	70	5.0	.3	12.4
Crab, including blue, Dungeness, rock and king:				
Cooked, steamed	93	17.3	1.9	.5
Crab, canned	101	17.4	2.5	1.1
Crab, deviled	188	11.4	9.4	13.3
Crab imperial	147	14.6	7.6	3.9
Crabapples, raw	68	.4	.3	17.8
Crackers:				
Animal	429	6.6	9.4	79.9
Butter	458	7.0	17.8	67.3
Cheese	479	11.2	21.3	60.4
Graham:				
Chocolate-coated	475	5.1	23.5	67.9
Plain	384	8.0	9.4	73.3
Sugar-honey coated	411	6.7	11.4	76.4
Saltines	433	9.0	12.0	71.5
Sandwich type, peanut-cheese	491	15.2	23.9	56.1
Soda	439	9.2	13.1	70.6
Whole-wheat	403	8.4	13.8	68.2
Cranberries:				
Raw	46	.4	.7	10.8
Dehydrated, uncooked	368	2.8	6.6	84.3
Cranberry juice cocktail, bottled (approx. 33% cranberry juice).	65	.1	.1	16.5

FOOD AND DESCRIPTION *(per 100 grams, edible portion)*	FOOD ENERGY *Calories*	PROTEIN *Grams*	FAT *Grams*	CARBO-HYDRATE *Grams*
Cranberry sauce, sweetened:				
Canned, strained	146	.1	.2	37.5
Home-prepared, unstrained ..	178	.2	.3	45.5
Cranberry-orange relish, uncooked	178	.4	.4	45.4
Crappie, white, raw	79	16.8	.8	0
Crayfish, freshwater; and spiny lobster; raw	72	14.6	.5	1.2
Cream, fluid:				
Half-and-half (cream and milk)	134	3.2	11.7	4.6
Light, coffee, or table	211	3.0	20.6	4.3
Light whipping	300	2.5	31.3	3.6
Heavy whipping......................	352	2.2	37.6	3.1
Cream substitutes, dried, containing—				
Cream, skim milk (calcium reduced) and lactose	508	8.5	26.7	61.3
Cream, skim milk, lactose, and sodium hexametaphosphate.	509	13.9	27.7	53.2
Cream puffs with custard filling	233	6.5	13.9	20.5
Cucumbers, raw:				
Not pared	15	.9	.1	3.4
Pared.......................................	14	.6	.1	3.2
Currants, raw:				
Black, European	54	1.7	.1	13.1
Red and white	50	1.4	.2	12.1
Dandelion greens:				
Raw..	45	2.7	.7	9.2
Cooked, boiled, drained..........	33	2.0	.6	6.4
Doughnuts:				
Cake type	391	4.6	18.6	51.4
Yeast-leavened........................	414	6.3	26.7	37.7
Duck, domesticated, raw:				
Total edible..............................	326	16.0	28.6	0
Flesh only................................	165	21.4	8.2	0
Duck, wild, raw:				
Total edible..............................	233	21.1	15.8	0
Flesh only................................	138	21.3	5.2	0

FOOD AND DESCRIPTION (per 100 grams, edible portion)	FOOD ENERGY Calories	PROTEIN Grams	FAT Grams	CARBO-HYDRATE Grams
Eclairs with custard filling and chocolate icing	239	6.2	13.6	23.2
Eel, American, raw	233	15.9	18.3	0
Eel, smoked	330	18.6	27.8	0
Eggs:				
Chicken:				
Raw:				
Whole, fresh, and frozen	163	12.9	11.5	.9
Whites, fresh, and frozen	51	10.9	Trace	.8
Yolks, fresh	348	16.0	30.6	.6
Yolks, frozen	312	15.4	26.9	.6
Yolks, frozen, sugared ..	315	14.3	24.0	9.9
Cooked:				
Fried	216	13.8	17.2	.3
Hard-cooked	163	12.9	11.5	.9
Omelet.............................	173	11.2	12.9	2.4
Poached............................	163	12.7	11.6	.8
Scrambled	173	11.2	12.9	2.4
Dried:				
Whole	592	47.0	41.2	4.1
Whole, stabilized (glucose reduced)	609	48.9	42.9	2.5
White, flakes....................	349	75.1	.2	5.3
White, powder	372	80.2	.2	5.7
Yolk..................................	664	33.2	56.6	2.5
Duck, whole, fresh, raw	191	13.3	14.5	.7
Goose, whole, fresh, raw	185	13.9	13.3	1.3
Turkey, whole, fresh, raw	170	13.1	11.8	1.7
Eggplant:				
Raw...	25	1.2	.2	5.6
Cooked, boiled, drained..........	19	1.0	.2	4.1
Elderberries, raw	72	2.6	(.5)	16.4
Endive (curly endive and escarole), raw	20	1.7	.1	4.1
Eulachon (smelt), raw	118	14.6	6.2	0
Farina:				
Enriched:				
Regular:				
Dry form..........................	371	11.4	.9	77.0
Cooked..............................	42	1.3	.1	8.7

FOOD AND DESCRIPTION *(per 100 grams, edible portion)*	FOOD ENERGY *Calories*	PROTEIN *Grams*	FAT *Grams*	CARBO-HYDRATE *Grams*
Quick-cooking:				
Dry form	362	11.4	.9	74.9
Cooked	43	1.3	.1	8.9
Instant-cooking:				
Dry form	362	11.4	.9	74.9
Cooked	55	1.7	.1	11.4
Unenriched, regular:				
Dry form	371	11.4	.9	77.0
Cooked	42	1.3	.1	8.7
Fats, cooking (vegetable fat) ..	884	0	100.	0
Fennel, common, leaves, raw..	28	2.8	.4	5.1
Figs:				
Raw	80	1.2	.3	20.3
Candied	299	3.5	.2	73.7
Canned, solids and liquid:				
Water pack, with or without artificial sweetener	48	.5	.2	12.4
Sirup pack:				
Light	65	.5	.2	16.8
Heavy	84	.5	.2	21.8
Extra heavy	103	.5	.2	26.7
Dried, uncooked	274	4.3	1.3	69.1
Filberts (hazelnuts)	634	12.6	62.4	16.7
Finnan haddie (smoked haddock)	103	23.2	.4	0
Fish cakes, cooked:				
Fried	172	14.7	8.0	9.3
Frozen, fried, reheated	270	9.2	17.9	17.2
Fish flakes, canned	111	24.7	.6	0
Fish flour:				
From whole fish	336	78.0	.3	0
From fillets	398	93.0	.1	0
From fillet waste	305	71.0	.2	0
Fish loaf, cooked	124	14.1	3.7	7.3
Fish sticks, frozen, cooked ..	176	16.6	8.9	6.5
Flatfishes (flounders, soles, and sanddabs), raw	79	16.7	.8	0
Flounder, cooked, baked	202	30.0	8.2	0
Frog legs, raw	73	16.4	.3	0

FOOD AND DESCRIPTION (per 100 grams, edible portion)	FOOD ENERGY Calories	PROTEIN Grams	FAT Grams	CARBO-HYDRATE Grams
Fruit cocktail, canned, solids and liquid:				
Water pack, with or without artificial sweetener	37	.4	.1	9.7
Sirup pack:				
Light	60	.4	.1	15.7
Heavy	76	.4	.1	19.7
Extra heavy	92	.4	.1	23.7
Fruit salad, canned, solids and liquid:				
Water pack, with or without artificial sweetener	35	.4	.1	9.1
Sirup pack:				
Light	59	.3	.1	15.5
Heavy	75	.3	.1	19.4
Extra heavy	90	.3	.1	23.4
Garlic, cloves, raw	137	6.2	.2	30.8
Gelatin, dry	335	85.6	.1	0
Gelatin dessert powder and desserts made from dessert powder:				
Dessert powder	371	9.4	0	88.0
Desserts, made with water:				
Plain	59	1.5	0	14.1
With fruit added	67	1.3	.1	16.4
Ginger root, crystallized (candied)	340	.3	.2	87.1
Ginger root, fresh	49	1.4	1.0	9.5
Gizzard:				
Chicken, all classes:				
Raw	113	20.1	2.7	.7
Cooked, simmered	148	27.0	3.3	.7
Goose, raw	139	21.4	5.3	0
Turkey, all classes:				
Raw	157	20.3	7.3	1.1
Cooked, simmered	196	26.8	8.6	1.1
Grapefruit:				
Raw:				
Pulp:				
Pink, red, white:				

FOOD AND DESCRIPTION *(per 100 grams, edible portion)*	FOOD ENERGY *Calories*	PROTEIN *Grams*	FAT *Grams*	CARBO-HYDRATE *Grams*
All varieties..................	41	.5	.1	10.6
Juice:				
Pink, red, and white:				
All varieties..................	39	.5	.1	9.2
Frozen concentrated juice:				
Unsweetened:				
Undiluted	145	1.9	.4	34.6
Diluted with 3 parts water, by volume	41	.5	.1	9.8
Sweetened:				
Undiluted	165	1.6	.3	40.2
Diluted with 3 parts water, by volume	47	.4	.1	11.4
Dehydrated juice (crystals):				
Dry form..............................	378	4.8	1.0	90.3
Prepared with water (1 lb. yields approx. 1 gal.)	40	.5	.1	9.6
Grapefruit juice and orange juice blended:				
Canned:				
Unsweetened	43	.6	.2	10.1
Sweetened............................	50	.5	.1	12.2
Frozen concentrate, unsweetened:				
Undiluted	157	2.1	.5	37.1
Diluted with 3 parts water, by volume	44	.6	.1	10.5
Grapefruit peel, candied	316	.4	.3	80.6
Grapes:				
Raw:				
American type (slip skin) as Concord, Delaware, Niagara, Catawba, and Scuppernong.	69	1.3	1.0	15.7
Grapejuice:				
Canned or bottled	66	.2	Trace	16.6
Frozen concentrate, sweetened:				
Undiluted	183	.6	Trace	46.3

FOOD AND DESCRIPTION (per 100 grams, edible portion)	FOOD ENERGY Calories	PROTEIN Grams	FAT Grams	CARBO-HYDRATE Grams
Diluted with 3 parts water, by volume	53	.2	Trace	13.3
Grapejuice drink, canned (approx. 30% grapejuice)	54	.1	Trace	13.8
Groundcherries (poha or cape-gooseberries), raw	53	1.9	.7	11.2
Grouper, including red, black, and speckled hind; raw	87	19.3	.5	0
Guavas, whole, raw:				
Common	62	.8	.6	15.0
Strawberry	65	1.0	.6	15.8
Guinea hen, raw:				
Total edible	156	23.1	6.4	0
Flesh and skin	158	23.4	6.4	0
Giblets	157	20.8	7.0	1.2
Haddock:				
Raw	79	18.3	.1	0
Cooked, fried	165	19.6	6.4	5.8
Smoked, canned or not canned	103	23.2	.4	0
Hake, including Pacific hake, squirrel hake, and silver hake or whiting; raw.	74	16.5	.4	0
Halibut, Atlantic and Pacific:				
Raw	100	20.9	1.2	0
Cooked, broiled	171	25.2	7.0	0
Smoked	224	20.8	15.0	0
Halibut, California, raw	97	19.8	1.4	0
Halibut, Greenland, raw	146	16.4	8.4	0
Ham croquette	251	16.3	15.1	11.7
Haws, scarlet, flesh and skin, raw	87	2.0	.7	20.8
Heart:				
Beef, lean:				
Raw	108	17.1	3.6	.7
Cooked, braised	188	31.3	5.7	.7
Beef, lean with visible fat:				
Raw	253	15.4	20.7	.1
Cooked, braised	372	25.8	29.0	.1
Calf:				
Raw	124	15.0	5.9	1.8

FOOD AND DESCRIPTION (per 100 grams, edible portion)	FOOD ENERGY Calories	PROTEIN Grams	FAT Grams	CARBO-HYDRATE Grams
Cooked, braised	208	27.8	9.1	1.8
Chicken, all classes:				
Raw	134	18.6	6.0	.1
Cooked, simmered	173	25.3	7.2	.1
Hog:				
Raw	113	16.8	4.4	.4
Cooked, braised	195	30.8	6.9	.3
Lamb:				
Raw	162	16.8	9.6	1.0
Cooked, braised	260	29.5	14.4	1.0
Turkey, all classes:				
Raw	171	16.2	11.2	.2
Cooked, simmered	216	22.6	13.2	.2
Herring.				
Raw:				
Atlantic	176	17.3	11.3	0
Pacific	98	17.5	2.6	0
Canned, solids and liquid:				
Plain	208	19.9	13.6	0
In tomato sauce	176	15.8	10.5	3.7
Pickled, Bismarck type	223	20.4	15.1	0
Salted or brined	218	19.0	15.2	0
Smoked:				
Bloaters	196	19.6	12.4	0
Hard	300	36.9	15.8	0
Kippered	211	22.2	12.9	0
Hickorynuts	673	13.2	68.7	12.8
Honey, strained or extracted	304	.3	0	82.3
Horseradish:				
Raw	87	3.2	.3	19.7
Prepared	38	1.3	.2	9.6
Hyacinth-beans, raw:				
Young pods	35	2.8	.3	7.3
Mature seeds, dry	338	22.2	1.5	61.0
Ice cream and frozen custard:				
Regular:				
Approximately 10% fat	193	4.5	10.6	20.8
Approximately 12% fat	207	4.0	12.5	20.6
Rich, approximately 16% fat	222	2.6	16.1	18.0
Ice cream cones	377	10.0	2.4	77.9

202   NUTRITION AND THE ATHLETE

FOOD AND DESCRIPTION (per 100 grams, edible portion)	FOOD ENERGY Calories	PROTEIN Grams	FAT Grams	CARBO-HYDRATE Grams
Ice milk	152	4.8	5.1	22.4
Ices, water, lime	78	.4	Trace	32.6
Inconnu (sheefish), raw	146	19.9	6.8	0
Jack mackerel, raw	143	21.6	5.6	0
Jackfruit, raw	98	1.3	.3	25.4
Jams and preserves	272	.6	.1	70.0
Jellies	273	.1	.1	70.6
Jerusalem-artichoke, raw		2.3	.1	16.7
Jujube, common (Chinese date):				
Raw	105	1.2	.2	27.6
Dried	287	3.7	1.1	73.6
Kale:				
Raw:				
Leaves, without stems, mid-ribs	53	(6.0)	(.8)	9.0
Leaves, including stems	38	4.2	.8	6.0
Cooked, boiled, drained:				
Leaves, without stems, mid-ribs	39	(4.5)	(.7)	6.1
Leaves, including stems	28	3.2	.7	4.0
Frozen:				
Not thawed	32	3.2	.5	5.5
Cooked, boiled, drained	31	3.0	.5	5.4
Kidneys:				
Beef:				
Raw	130	15.4	6.7	.9
Cooked, braised	252	33.0	12.0	.8
Calf, raw	113	16.6	4.6	.1
Hog, raw	106	16.3	3.6	1.1
Lamb, raw	105	16.8	3.3	.9
Kingfish; southern, gulf, and northern (whiting); raw.	105	18.3	3.0	0
Lake herring (cisco), raw	96	17.7	2.3	0
Lake trout, raw	168	18.3	10.0	0
Lake trout (siscowet), raw:				
Less than 6.5 lbs., round weight	241	14.3	19.9	0
6.5 lbs. and over, round weight	524	7.9	54.4	0

FOOD AND DESCRIPTION *(per 100 grams, edible portion)*	FOOD ENERGY Calories	PROTEIN Grams	FAT Grams	CARBO-HYDRATE Grams
Lamb:				
Composite of cuts (leg, loin, rib, and shoulder) trimmed to retail level:				
Prime grade (72% lean, 28% fat)	310	15.4	27.1	0
Choice grade (77% lean, 23% fat)	263	16.5	21.3	0
Good grade (79% lean, 21% fat)	247	16.8	19.4	0
Lard.................................	902	0	100	0
Leeks, bulb and lower leaf portion, raw	52	2.2	.3	11.2
Lemons, raw:				
Peeled fruit	27	1.1	.3	8.2
Fruit, including peel	20	1.2	.3	10.7
Lemon juice:				
Raw...	25	.5	.2	8.0
Canned or bottled, unsweetened	23	.4	.1	7.6
Frozen, unsweetened:				
Single-strength juice	22	.4	.2	7.2
Concentrate	116	2.3	.9	37.4
Lemon peel:				
Raw...		1.5	.3	16.0
Candied....................................	316	.4	.3	80.6
Lemonade concentrate, frozen:				
Undiluted	195	.2	.1	51.1
Diluted with 4 1/3 parts water, by volume	44	.1	Trace	11.4
Lentils, mature seeds, dry:				
Whole:				
Raw.......................................	340	24.7	1.1	60.1
Cooked	106	7.8	Trace	19.3
Split, without seed coat, raw	345	24.7	.9	61.8
Lettuce, raw:				
Butterhead varieties such as Boston types and Bibb	14	1.2	.2	2.5

FOOD AND DESCRIPTION (per 100 grams, edible portion)	FOOD ENERGY Calories	PROTEIN Grams	FAT Grams	CARBO-HYDRATE Grams
Cos, or romaine, such as Dark Green and White Paris.	18	1.3	.3	3.5
Crisphead varieties such as Iceberg, New York, and Great Lakes strains.	13	.9	.1	2.9
Looseleaf, or bunching varieties, such as Grand Rapids, Salad Bowl, Simpson.	18	1.3	.3	3.5
Limes, acid type, raw	28	.7	.2	9.5
Lime juice:				
Raw...	26	.3	.1	9.0
Canned or bottled, unsweetened	26	.3	.1	9.0
Limeade concentrate, frozen:				
Undiluted	187	.2	.1	49.5
Diluted with 4 1/3 parts water, by volume	41	Trace	Trace	11.0
Lingcod, raw	84	17.9	.8	0
Liver:				
Beef:				
Raw.......................................	140	19.9	3.8	5.3
Cooked, fried	229	26.4	10.6	5.3
Calf:				
Raw.......................................	140	19.2	4.7	4.1
Cooked, fried	261	29.5	13.2	4.0
Chicken, all classes:				
Raw.......................................	129	19.7	3.7	2.9
Cooked, simmered	165	26.5	4.4	3.1
Goose, raw	182	16.5	10.0	5.4
Hog:				
Raw.......................................	131	20.6	3.7	2.6
Cooked, fried	241	29.9	11.5	2.5
Lamb:				
Raw.......................................	136	21.0	3.9	2.9
Cooked, broiled....................	261	32.3	12.4	2.8
Turkey, all classes:				
Raw.......................................	138	21.2	4.0	2.9
Cooked, simmered	174	27.9	4.8	3.1
Lobster, northern:				
Raw, whole..............................	91	16.9	1.9	0.5
Canned or cooked	95	18.7	1.5	.3

FOOD AND DESCRIPTION *(per 100 grams, edible portion)*	FOOD ENERGY *Calories*	PROTEIN *Grams*	FAT *Grams*	CARBO- HYDRATE *Grams*
Lobster Newburg....................	194	18.5	10.6	5.1
Lobster salad............................	110	10.1	6.4	2.3
Loganberries:				
Raw...	62	1.0	.6	14.9
Canned, solids and liquid:				
Water pack, with or without artificial sweetener	40	.7	.4	9.4
Juice pack............................	54	.7	.5	12.7
Sirup pack:				
Light	70	.7	.4	17.2
Heavy	89	.6	.4	22.2
Extra heavy	108	.6	.4	27.2
Macadamia nuts......................	691	7.8	71.6	15.9
Macaroni:				
Enriched:				
Dry form..............................	369	12.5	1.2	75.2
Cooked, firm stage (8–10 min.)	148	5.0	.5	30.1
Cooked, tender stage (14–20 min.)	111	3.4	.4	23.0
Unenriched:				
Dry form..............................	369	12.5	1.2	75.2
Cooked, firm stage (8–10 min.)	148	5.0	.5	30.1
Cooked, tender stage (14–20 min.)	111	3.4	.4	23.0
Macaroni and cheese:				
Baked, made from home recipe	215	8.4	11.1	20.1
Canned	95	3.9	4.0	10.7
Mackerel, Atlantic:				
Raw...	191	19.0	12.2	0
Canned, solids and liquid	183	19.3	11.1	0
Cooked, broiled with butter or margarine	236	21.8	15.8	0
Mackerel, Pacific:				
Raw...	159	21.9	7.3	0
Canned, solids and liquid	180	21.1	10.0	0
Mackerel:				
Salted	305	18.5	25.1	0
Smoked	219	23.8	13.0	0

FOOD AND DESCRIPTION *(per 100 grams, edible portion)*	FOOD ENERGY Calories	PROTEIN Grams	FAT Grams	CARBO-HYDRATE Grams
Malt, dry...................................	368	13.1	1.9	77.4
Malt extract, dried	367	6.0	Trace	89.2
Mamey (mammeeapple), raw ..	51	.5	.5	12.5
Mangos, raw	66	.7	.4	16.8
Margarine	720	.6	81.	.4
Marmalade, citrus	257	.5	.1	70.1
Milk, cow:				
Fluid (pasteurized and raw):				
Whole:				
3.5% fat.............................	65	3.5	3.5	4.9
3.7% fat.............................	66	3.5	3.7	4.9
Skim	36	3.6	.1	5.1
Partially skimmed with 2% nonfat milk solids added.	59	4.2	2.0	6.0
Canned:				
Evaporated (unsweetened)	137	7.0	7.9	9.7
Condensed (sweetened)	321	8.1	8.7	54.3
Dry:				
Whole	502	26.4	27.5	38.2
Skim (nonfat solids), regular	363	35.9	.8	52.3
Skim (nonfat solids), instant	359	35.8	.7	51.6
Malted:				
Dry powder	410	14.7	8.3	70.8
Beverage...........................	104	4.7	4.4	11.7
Chocolate drink, fluid, commercial:				
Made with skim milk..........	76	3.3	2.3	10.9
Made with whole (3.5% fat) milk	85	3.4	3.4	11.0
Chocolate beverages, homemade:				
Hot chocolate	95	3.3	5.0	10.4
Hot cocoa	97	3.8	4.6	10.9
Milk, goat, fluid......................	67	3.2	4.0	4.6
Milk, human, U.S. samples	77	1.1	4.0	9.5
Milk, reindeer	234	10.8	19.6	4.1
Millet, proso (broomcorn, hog-millet), whole-grain	327	9.9	2.9	72.9

FOOD AND DESCRIPTION (per 100 grams, edible portion)	FOOD ENERGY Calories	PROTEIN Grams	FAT Grams	CARBO-HYDRATE Grams
Molasses, cane:				
First extraction or light	252	—	—	65.
Second extraction or medium	232	—	—	60.
Third extraction or blackstrap	213	—	—	55.
Barbados.................................	271	—	—	70.
Muffins, baked from home recipes:				
Plain, made with—				
Enriched flour	294	7.8	10.1	42.3
Unenriched flour	294	7.8	10.1	42.3
Other, made with enriched flour:				
Blueberry	281	7.3	9.3	41.9
Bran	261	7.7	9.8	43.1
Corn, made with—				
Enriched degermed corn-meal	314	7.1	10.1	48.1
Whole-ground cornmeal..	288	7.2	10.3	42.5
Muffin mixes, corn, and muffins baked from mixes:				
Mix, dry form, with enriched flour	417	6.2	11.5	71.8
Muffins, made with egg, milk	324	6.9	10.6	50.0
Mix, dry form, with cake flour, nonfat dry milk	409	6.2	10.7	71.6
Muffins, made with egg, water	297	4.5	7.8	51.9
Mushrooms:				
Agaricus campestris, cultivated commercially:				
Raw	28	2.7	.3	4.4
Canned, solids and liquid ..	17	1.9	.1	2.4
Other edible species, raw	35	1.9	.6	6.5
Muskellunge, raw....................	109	20.2	2.5	0
Muskmelons:				
Raw:				
Cantaloupes, other netted varieties	30	.7	.1	7.5

FOOD AND DESCRIPTION *(per 100 grams, edible portion)*	FOOD ENERGY Calories	PROTEIN Grams	FAT Grams	CARBO-HYDRATE Grams
Casaba (Golden Beauty)	27	1.2	Trace	6.5
Honeydew............................	33	.8	.3	7.7
Frozen:				
Melon balls (cantaloupe and honeydew) in sirup, not thawed.	62	.6	.1	15.7
Muskrat, cooked, roasted........	153	27.2	4.1	0
Mussels, Atlantic and Pacific, raw:				
Meat and liquid	66	9.6	1.4	3.1
Meat only	95	14.4	2.2	3.3
Mussels, Pacific, canned, drained solids	114	18.2	3.3	1.5
Mustard greens:				
Raw...	31	3.0	.5	5.6
Cooked, boiled, drained..........	23	2.2	.4	4.0
Frozen:				
Not thawed...........................	20	2.3	.4	3.2
Cooked, boiled, drained	20	2.2	.4	3.1
Mustard spinach (tendergreen):				
Raw...	22	2.2	.3	3.9
Cooked, boiled, drained..........	16	1.7	.2	2.8
Mustard, prepared:				
Brown	91	5.9	6.3	5.3
Yellow.....................................	75	4.7	4.4	6.4
Nectarines, raw......................	64	.6	Trace	17.1
New Zealand spinach:				
Raw...	19	2.2	.3	3.1
Cooked, boiled, drained..........	13	1.7	.2	2.1
Noodles, egg noodles:				
Enriched:				
Dry form.............................	388	12.8	4.6	72.0
Cooked	125	4.1	1.5	23.3
Unenriched:				
Dry form.............................	388	12.8	4.6	72.0
Cooked	125	4.1	1.5	23.3
Noodles, chow mein, canned	489	13.2	23.5	58.0
Nuts. See individual kinds.				

The Composition of Foods

FOOD AND DESCRIPTION (per 100 grams, edible portion)	FOOD ENERGY Calories	PROTEIN Grams	FAT Grams	CARBO-HYDRATE Grams
Oat products used mainly as hot breakfast cereals:				
Oat cereal with toasted wheat germ and soy grits:				
Dry form..............................	382	20.5	9.0	58.6
Cooked	62	3.3	1.5	9.5
Oat flakes, maple-flavored, instant-cooking:				
Dry form..............................	384	14.6	4.2	72.3
Cooked	69	2.6	.8	13.0
Oat granules, maple-flavored, quick-cooking:				
Dry form..............................	383	14.8	4.0	72.5
Cooked	60	2.3	.6	11.4
Oat and wheat cereal:				
Dry form..............................	364	14.7	5.0	68.3
Cooked	65	2.6	.9	12.1
Oatmeal or rolled oats:				
Dry form..............................	390	14.2	7.4	68.2
Cooked	55	2.0	1.0	9.7
Oat products used mainly as ready-to-eat breakfast cereals:				
Oats, shredded, with protein and other added nutrients.	379	18.8	2.1	72.0
Oats (with or without corn), puffed, added nutrients	397	11.9	5.5	75.2
Oats (with or without corn, wheat), puffed, added nutrients, sugar-covered.	396	6.7	3.4	85.6
Oats (with soy flour and rice), flaked, added nutrients	397	14.9	5.7	70.7
Ocean perch, Atlantic (redfish):				
Raw......................................	88	18.0	1.2	0
Cooked, fried	227	19.0	13.3	6.8
Frozen, breaded, fried, reheated	319	18.9	18.9	16.5

FOOD AND DESCRIPTION *(per 100 grams, edible portion)*	FOOD ENERGY *Calories*	PROTEIN *Grams*	FAT *Grams*	CARBO-HYDRATE *Grams*
Ocean perch, Pacific, raw	95	19.0	1.5	0
Octopus, raw	73	15.3	.8	0
Oils, salad or cooking	884	0	100.	0
Okra:				
Raw...	36	2.4	.3	7.6
Cooked, boiled, drained..........	29	2.0	.3	6.0
Frozen, cuts and pods:				
Not thawed...........................	39	2.3	.1	9.0
Cooked, boiled, drained	38	2.2	.1	8.8
Olives, pickled; canned or bottled:				
Green	116	1.4	12.7	1.3
Ripe:				
Ascolano (extra large, mammoth, giant, jumbo)	129	1.1	13.8	2.6
Manzanilla (small, medium, large, extra large)	129	1.1	13.8	2.6
Mission (small, medium, large, extra large)	184	1.2	20.1	3.2
Sevillano (giant, jumbo, colossal, supercolossal)	93	1.1	9.5	2.7
Ripe, salt-cured, oil-coated, Greek style	338	2.2	35.8	8.7
Omelet. See Eggs, omelet				
Onions, mature (dry):				
Raw...	38	1.5	.1	8.7
Cooked, boiled, drained..........	29	1.2	.1	6.5
Dehydrated, flaked	350	8.7	1.3	82.1
Onions, young green (bunching varieties), raw:				
Bulb and entire top................	36	1.5	.2	8.2
Bulb and white portion of top	45	1.1	.2	10.5
Tops only (green portion)	27	1.6	.4	5.5
Onions, Welsh, raw	34	1.9	.4	6.5
Opossum, cooked, roasted	221	30.2	10.2	0
Oranges, raw:				
Peeled fruit:				
All commercial varieties	49	1.0	.2	12.2

FOOD AND DESCRIPTION (per 100 grams, edible portion)	FOOD ENERGY Calories	PROTEIN Grams	FAT Grams	CARBO-HYDRATE Grams
California:				
Navels (winter oranges)	51	1.3	.1	12.7
Valencias (summer oranges)	51	1.2	.3	12.4
Florida:				
All commercial varieties	47	.7	(.2)	12.0
Fruit, including peel (California Valencias)	40	1.3	.3	15.5
Orange juice:				
Raw:				
All commercial varieties	45	.7	.2	10.4
California:				
Navels (winter oranges)	48	1.0	.1	11.3
Valencias (summer oranges)	47	1.0	.3	10.5
Florida:				
All commercial varieties	43	.6	.2	10.0
Early and midseason oranges (Hamlin, Parson Brown, Pineapple).	40	.5	.2	9.3
Late season (Valencias)..	45	.6	.2	10.5
Temple.............................	54	(.5)	(.2)	12.9
Canned:				
Unsweetened	48	.8	.2	11.2
Sweetened............................	52	.7	.2	12.2
Canned concentrate, unsweetened:				
Undiluted	223	4.1	1.3	50.7
Diluted with 5 parts water, by volume	46	.8	.3	10.3
Frozen concentrate, unsweetened:				
Undiluted	158	2.3	.2	38.0
Diluted with 3 parts water, by volume	45	.7	.1	10.7
Oysters:				
Raw, meat only:				
Eastern	66	8.4	1.8	3.4

FOOD AND DESCRIPTION *(per 100 grams, edible portion)*	FOOD ENERGY *Calories*	PROTEIN *Grams*	FAT *Grams*	CARBO-HYDRATE *Grams*
Pacific and Western (Olympia)............................	91	10.6	2.2	6.4
Cooked, fried	239	8.6	13.9	18.6
Canned, solids and liquid	76	8.5	2.2	4.9
Frozen, solids and liquid........	—	6.1	—	—
Oyster stew:				
Commercial, frozen:				
Condensed.............................	102	4.6	6.3	6.9
Prepared with equal volume of water	51	2.3	3.2	3.4
Prepared with equal volume of milk	84	4.2	4.9	5.9
Home-prepared:				
1 part oysters to 2 parts milk by volume	97	5.2	6.4	4.5
1 part oysters to 3 parts milk by volume	86	4.9	5.3	4.7
Pancakes, baked from home recipe, made with—				
Enriched flour	231	7.1	7.0	34.1
Unenriched flour	231	7.1	7.0	34.1
Pancake and waffle mixes and pancakes baked from mixes:				
Plain and buttermilk:				
Mix (pancake and waffle), with enriched flour, dry form.	356	8.6	1.8	75.7
Pancakes:				
Made with milk............	202	6.1	5.6	31.9
Made with egg, milk ..	225	7.2	7.3	32.4
Mix (pancake and waffle), with unenriched flour, dry form.	356	8.6	1.8	75.7
Pancakes:				
Made with milk............	202	6.1	5.6	31.9
Made with egg, milk ..	225	7.2	7.3	32.4
Buckwheat and other cereal flours:				
Mix, dry form......................	328	10.5	1.9	70.3

FOOD AND DESCRIPTION *(per 100 grams, edible portion)*	FOOD ENERGY *Calories*	PROTEIN *Grams*	FAT *Grams*	CARBO-HYDRATE *Grams*
Pancakes, made with egg, milk	200	6.8	9.1	23.8
Pancreas, raw:				
Beef:				
Very fat	357	11.8	34.	0
Fat..	316	12.8	29.	0
Medium-fat	283	13.5	25.	0
Thin	217	14.9	17.	0
Lean only, adhering fat removed	141	17.6	7.3	0
Calf	161	19.2	8.8	0
Hog (hog sweetbread).............	242	14.7	19.9	0
Papaws, common, North American type, raw	85	5.2	.9	16.8
Papayas, raw	39	.6	.1	10.0
Parsley, common garden (plain) and curled-leaf varieties, raw.	44	3.6	.6	8.5
Parsnips:				
Raw..	76	1.7	.5	17.5
Cooked, boiled, drained..........	66	1.5	.5	14.9
Pastinas, enriched, dry form:				
Egg	383	12.9	4.1	71.8
Vegetable:				
Carrot	371	11.9	1.6	75.7
Spinach	368	12.4	1.6	74.8
Pâté de foie gras, canned	462	11.4	43.8	4.8
Peaches:				
Raw..	38	.6	.1	9.7
Canned, solids and liquid:				
Water pack, with or without artificial sweetener	31	.4	.1	8.1
Juice pack.............................	45	.6	.1	11.6
Sirup pack:				
Light	58	.4	.1	15.1
Heavy	78	.4	.1	20.1
Extra heavy	97	.4	.1	25.1
Dehydrated, sulfured, nugget-type and pieces:				

FOOD AND DESCRIPTION (per 100 grams, edible portion)	FOOD ENERGY Calories	PROTEIN Grams	FAT Grams	CARBO-HYDRATE Grams
Uncooked	340	4.8	(.9)	88.0
Cooked, fruit and liquid, with added sugar	121	1.1	(.2)	31.3
Dried, sulfured:				
Uncooked	262	3.1	.7	68.3
Cooked, fruit and liquid:				
Without added sugar......	82	1.0	.2	21.4
With added sugar............	119	.9	.2	30.8
Frozen, sliced, sweetened, not thawed	88	.4	.1	22.6
Peach nectar, canned (approx. 40% fruit)	48	.2	Trace	12.4
Peanuts:				
Raw, with skins.......................	564	26.0	47.5	18.6
Raw, without skins	568	26.3	48.4	17.6
Boiled	376	15.5	31.5	14.5
Roasted, with skins................	582	26.2	48.7	20.6
Roasted and salted	585	26.0	49.8	18.8
Peanut butters made with—				
Small amounts of added fat, salt	581	27.8	49.4	17.2
Small amounts of added fat, sweetener, salt	582	25.5	49.5	19.5
Moderate amounts of added fat, sweetener, salt	589	25.2	50.6	18.8
Peanut spread...........................	601	20.3	52.1	22.0
Peanut flour, defatted	371	47.9	9.2	31.5
Pears:				
Raw, including skin................	61	.7	.4	15.3
Candied.....................................	303	1.3	.6	75.9
Canned, solids and liquid:				
Water pack, with or without artificial sweetener	32	.2	.2	8.3
Juice pack	46	.3	.3	11.8
Sirup pack:				
Light	61	.2	.2	15.6
Heavy	76	.2	.2	19.6
Extra heavy	92	.2	.2	23.6
Dried, sulfured:				
Uncooked	268	3.1	1.8	67.3

FOOD AND DESCRIPTION *(per 100 grams, edible portion)*	FOOD ENERGY Calories	PROTEIN Grams	FAT Grams	CARBO-HYDRATE Grams
Cooked, fruit and liquid:				
Without added sugar......	126	1.5	.8	31.7
With added sugar............	151	1.3	.8	38.0
Pear nectar, canned (approx. 40% fruit)	52	.3	.2	13.2
Peas, edible-podded:				
Raw..	53	3.4	.2	12.0
Cooked, boiled, drained..........	43	2.9	.2	9.5
Peas, green, immature:				
Raw..	84	6.3	.4	14.4
Cooked, boiled, drained..........	71	5.4	.4	12.1
Canned:				
Alaska (Early or June peas):				
Regular pack:				
Solids and liquid..........	66	3.5	.3	12.5
Drained solids..............	88	4.7	.4	16.8
Drained liquid..............	26	1.3	Trace	5.2
Special dietary pack (low-sodium):				
Solids and liquid..........	55	3.6	.3	9.8
Drained solids..............	78	4.8	.4	14.3
Drained liquid..............	22	1.4	Trace	4.1
Sweet (sweet wrinkled peas, sugar peas):				
Regular pack:				
Solids and liquid..............	57	3.4	0.3	10.4
Drained solids..................	80	4.6	.4	15.0
Drained liquid..................	22	1.3	Trace	4.3
Special dietary pack (low-sodium):				
Solids and liquid..............	47	3.3	.3	8.2
Drained solids..................	72	4.4	.4	13.0
Drained liquid..................	18	1.3	Trace	3.4
Frozen:				
Not thawed..........................	73	5.4	.3	12.8
Cooked, boiled, drained......	68	5.1	.3	11.8
Peas, mature seeds, dry:				
Whole:				
Raw.......................................	340	24.1	1.3	60.3

FOOD AND DESCRIPTION *(per 100 grams, edible portion)*	FOOD ENERGY Calories	PROTEIN Grams	FAT Grams	CARBO-HYDRATE Grams
Split, without seed coat:				
Raw	348	24.2	1.0	62.7
Cooked	115	8.0	.3	20.8
Peas and carrots, frozen:				
Not thawed	55	3.3	.3	10.4
Cooked, boiled, drained..........	53	3.2	.3	10.1
Pecans.....................................	687	9.2	71.2	14.6
Peppers, hot, chili:				
Immature, green:				
Raw pods, excluding seeds	37	1.3	.2	9.1
Canned:				
Pods, excluding seeds; solids and liquid	25	.9	.1	6.1
Chili sauce........................	20	.7	.1	5.0
Mature, red:				
Raw:				
Pods, including seeds......	93	3.7	2.3	18.1
Pods, excluding seeds	65	2.3	.4	15.8
Canned, chili sauce	21	.9	.6	3.9
Dried:				
Pods..................................	321	12.9	9.1	59.8
Chili powder with added seasoning	340	14.3	12.4	56.5
Peppers, sweet, garden varieties:				
Immature, green:				
Raw	22	1.2	.2	4.8
Cooked:				
Boiled, drained	18	1.0	.2	3.8
Stuffed with beef and crumbs	170	13.0	5.5	16.8
Mature, red, raw	31	1.4	.3	7.1
Perch, white, raw....................	118	19.3	4.0	0
Perch, yellow, raw.................	91	19.5	.9	0
Persimmons, raw:				
Japanese or kaki	77	.7	.4	19.7
Native.....................................	127	.8	.4	33.5
Pheasant, raw:				
Total edible.............................	151	24.3	5.2	0
Flesh and skin	152	24.7	5.2	0

FOOD AND DESCRIPTION *(per 100 grams, edible portion)*	FOOD ENERGY *Calories*	PROTEIN *Grams*	FAT *Grams*	CARBO- HYDRATE *Grams*
Flesh only...............................	162	23.6	6.8	0
Giblets......................................	139	20.8	4.9	1.6
Pickerel, chain, raw	84	18.7	.5	0
Pickles:				
Cucumber:				
Dill..	11	.7	.2	2.2
Fresh (as bread-and-butter pickles)	73	.9	.2	17.9
Sour......................................	10	.5	.2	2.0
Sweet....................................	146	.7	.4	36.5
Chowchow (Cucumber with added cauliflower, onion, mustard):				
Sour......................................	29	1.4	1.3	4.1
Sweet....................................	116	1.5	.9	27.0
Relish, finely cut or chopped:				
Sour......................................	19	(.7)	(.9)	(2.7)
Sweet....................................	138	.5	.6	34.0
Pies:				
Baked, piecrust made with unenriched flour:				
Apple....................................	256	2.2	11.1	38.1
Banana custard	221	4.5	9.3	30.7
Blackberry	243	2.6	11.0	34.4
Blueberry	242	2.4	10.8	34.9
Butterscotch........................	267	4.4	11.0	38.3
Cherry..................................	261	2.6	11.3	38.4
Chocolate chiffon	328	6.8	15.3	43.7
Chocolate meringue...........	252	4.8	12.0	33.5
Coconut custard..................	235	6.0	12.5	24.9
Custard	218	6.1	11.1	23.4
Lemon chiffon......................	313	7.0	12.6	43.8
Lemon meringue	255	3.7	10.2	37.7
Mince....................................	271	2.5	11.5	41.2
Peach....................................	255	2.5	10.7	38.2
Pecan....................................	418	5.1	22.9	51.3
Pineapple	253	2.2	10.7	38.1
Pineapple chiffon	288	6.6	12.1	39.1
Pineapple custard	220	4.0	8.7	32.1
Pumpkin	211	4.0	11.2	24.5

FOOD AND DESCRIPTION (per 100 grams, edible portion)	FOOD ENERGY Calories	PROTEIN Grams	FAT Grams	CARBO- HYDRATE Grams
Raisin	270	2.6	10.7	43.0
Rhubarb	253	2.5	10.7	38.2
Strawberry	198	1.9	7.9	30.9
Sweetpotato	213	4.5	11.3	23.7
Frozen in unbaked form:				
Apple:				
Unbaked	210	1.6	8.3	33.2
Baked	254	1.9	10.1	40.0
Cherry:				
Unbaked	256	1.9	10.6	39.0
Baked	291	2.2	12.0	44.4
Coconut custard:				
Unbaked	205	5.2	8.5	27.1
Baked	249	6.0	12.0	29.5
Pie mix, coconut custard, and pie baked from mix:				
Mix, filling and piecrust, dry form	470	3.3	20.0	70.6
Pie prepared with egg yolk and milk, baked	203	4.3	7.9	29.1
Piecrust or plain pastry, made with—				
Enriched flour:				
Unbaked	464	5.7	31.0	40.7
Baked	500	6.1	33.4	43.8
Unenriched flour:				
Unbaked	464	5.7	31.0	40.7
Baked	500	6.1	33.4	43.8
Piecrust mix (including stick form) and piecrust baked from mix:				
Mix, dry form	522	7.2	32.7	49.5
Piecrust, prepared with water, baked	464	6.4	29.1	44.0
Pigeonpeas, raw:				
Immature seeds......................	117	7.2	.6	21.3
Mature seeds, dry	342	20.4	1.4	63.7
Pigs' feet, pickled	199	16.7	14.8	0
Pike, blue, raw	90	19.1	.9	0
Pike, northern, raw	88	18.3	1.1	0

FOOD AND DESCRIPTION (per 100 grams, edible portion)	FOOD ENERGY Calories	PROTEIN Grams	FAT Grams	CARBO-HYDRATE Grams
Pike, walleye, raw	93	19.3	1.2	0
Pilinuts	669	11.4	71.1	8.4
Pimientos, canned, solids and liquid	27	.9	.5	5.8
Pineapple:				
Raw..	52	0.4	0.2	13.7
Candied.....................................	316	.8	.4	80.0
Canned, solids and liquid:				
Water pack, all styles except crushed, with or without artificial sweetener.	39	.3	.1	10.2
Juice pack, all styles	58	.4	.1	15.1
Sirup pack, all styles:				
Light	59	.3	.1	15.4
Heavy	74	.3	.1	19.4
Extra heavy	90	.3	.1	23.4
Frozen chunks, sweetened, not thawed	85	.4	.1	22.2
Pineapple juice:				
Canned, unsweetened	55	.4	.1	13.5
Frozen concentrate, unsweetened:				
Undiluted	179	1.3	.1	44.3
Diluted with 3 parts water, by volume	52	.4	Trace	12.8
Pineapple juice and grapefruit juice drink, canned (approx. 40% fruit juices)	54	.2	Trace	13.6
Pineapple juice and orange juice drink, canned (approx. 40% fruit juices)	54	.2	.1	13.5
Pinenuts:				
Pignolias....................................	552	31.1	47.4	11.6
Piñon...	635	13.0	60.5	20.5
Pistachionuts	594	19.3	53.7	19.0
Pitanga (Surinam-cherry), raw	51	.8	.4	12.5
Pizza, with cheese:				
From home recipe, baked:				

FOOD AND DESCRIPTION (per 100 grams, edible portion)	FOOD ENERGY Calories	PROTEIN Grams	FAT Grams	CARBO-HYDRATE Grams
With cheese topping	236	12.0	8.3	28.3
With sausage topping	234	7.8	9.3	29.6
Chilled:				
Partially baked....................	208	7.8	5.8	30.9
Baked	245	9.2	6.8	36.3
Frozen:				
Partially baked....................	229	8.9	6.6	33.1
Baked	245	9.5	7.1	35.4
Plantain (baking banana), raw	119	1.1	.4	31.2
Plate dinners, frozen, commercial, unheated:				
Beef pot roast, whole oven-browned potatoes, peas, and corn.	106	13.1	3.2	6.1
Chicken, fried; mashed potatoes; mixed vegetables (carrots, peas, corn, beans).	173	12.8	8.5	11.3
Meat loaf with tomato sauce, mashed potatoes, and peas.	131	8.0	6.7	9.8
Turkey, sliced; mashed potatoes; peas	112	8.4	3.0	12.7
Plums:				
Raw:				
Damson.................................	66	.5	Trace	17.8
Japanese and hybrid	48	.5	.2	12.3
Prune-type	75	.8	.2	19.7
Canned, solids and liquid:				
Greengage, water pack, with or without artificial sweetener.	33	.4	.1	8.6
Purple (Italian prunes):				
Water pack, with or without artificial sweetener.	46	.4	.2	11.9
Sirup pack:				
Light	63	.4	.1	16.6
Heavy	83	.4	.1	21.6
Extra heavy	102	.4	.1	26.7

FOOD AND DESCRIPTION (per 100 grams, edible portion)	FOOD ENERGY Calories	PROTEIN Grams	FAT Grams	CARBO-HYDRATE Grams
Pollock:				
Raw..	95	20.4	.9	0
Cooked, creamed	128	13.9	5.9	4.0
Pomegranate pulp, raw	63	.5	.3	16.4
Pompano, raw	166	18.8	9.5	0
Popcorn:				
Unpopped	362	11.9	4.7	72.1
Popped:				
Plain	386	12.7	5.0	76.7
Oil and salt added	456	9.8	21.8	59.1
Sugar-coated........................	383	6.1	3.5	85.4
Popovers, baked (from home recipe with enriched flour).	224	8.8	9.2	25.8
Porgy and scup, raw	112	19.0	3.4	0
Pork, fresh:				
Carcass, raw:				
Fat class:				
Total edible (41% lean, 59% fat)	553	9.1	57.0	0
Separable lean	185	17.3	12.3	0
Separable fat	784	3.2	85.4	0
Medium-fat class:				
Total edible (47% lean, 53% fat)	513	10.2	52.0	0
Separable lean	171	17.8	10.5	0
Separable fat	770	3.5	83.7	0
Thin class:				
Total edible (53% lean, 47% fat)	472	11.2	47.0	0
Separable lean	156	18.3	8.6	0
Separable fat	755	3.7	81.9	0
Retail cuts, trimmed to retail level:				
Ham:				
Fat class:				
Total edible:				
Raw (72% lean, 28% fat)	327	15.2	29.1	0
Cooked, roasted (72% lean, 28% fat)	394	21.9	33.3	0

FOOD AND DESCRIPTION (per 100 grams, edible portion)	FOOD ENERGY Calories	PROTEIN Grams	FAT Grams	CARBO-HYDRATE Grams
Separable lean:				
Raw	160	19.7	8.4	0
Cooked, roasted	225	29.3	11.1	0
Separable fat:				
Raw	755	4.0	81.8	0
Medium-fat class:				
Total edible:				
Raw (74% lean, 26% fat)	308	15.9	26.6	0
Cooked, roasted (74% lean, 26% fat)	374	23.0	30.6	0
Separable lean:				
Raw	153	20.0	7.5	0
Cooked, roasted	217	29.7	10.0	0
Separable fat:				
Raw	746	4.3	80.7	0
Thin class:				
Total edible:				
Raw (77% lean, 23% fat)	281	16.7	23.2	0
Cooked, roasted (77% lean, 23% fat)	346	24.2	26.9	0
Separable lean:				
Raw	147	20.4	6.6	0
Cooked, roasted	210	30.2	9.0	0
Separable fat:				
Raw	737	4.6	79.5	0
Loin:				
Fat class:				
Total edible:				
Raw (76% lean, 24% fat)	323	16.4	28.0	0
Cooked, roasted (76% lean, 24% fat)	387	23.5	31.8	0
Cooked, broiled (68% lean, 32% fat)	418	23.5	35.2	0
Separable lean:				
Raw	189	20.1	11.4	0
Cooked, roasted	254	29.4	14.2	0
Cooked, broiled	270	30.6	15.4	0

FOOD AND DESCRIPTION *(per 100 grams, edible portion)*	FOOD ENERGY *Calories*	PROTEIN *Grams*	FAT *Grams*	CARBO-HYDRATE *Grams*
Separable fat:				
Raw	739	4.8	79.7	0
Medium-fat class:				
Total edible:				
Raw (80% lean, 20% fat)	298	17.1	24.9	0
Cooked, roasted (80% lean, 20% fat)	362	24.5	28.5	0
Cooked, broiled (72% lean, 28% fat)	391	24.7	31.7	0
Separable lean:				
Raw	189	20.1	11.4	0
Cooked, roasted	254	29.4	14.2	0
Cooked, broiled	270	30.6	15.4	0
Separable fat:				
Raw	723	5.2	77.7	0
Thin class:				
Total edible:				
Raw (85% lean, 15% fat)	268	17.9	21.2	0
Cooked, roasted (85% lean, 15% fat)	333	25.8	24.7	0
Spareribs:				
Fat class:				
Total edible:				
Raw	390	13.7	36.8	0
Cooked, braised........	467	19.7	42.5	0
Medium-fat class:				
Total edible:				
Raw	361	14.5	33.2	0
Cooked, braised........	440	20.8	38.9	0
Thin class:				
Total edible:				
Raw	331	15.3	29.5	0
Cooked, braised........	410	21.9	35.1	0
Pork, cured, canned:				
Ham, contents of can	193	18.3	12.3	.9
Pork and gravy, canned (90% pork, 10% gravy)	256	16.4	17.8	6.3

FOOD AND DESCRIPTION *(per 100 grams, edible portion)*	FOOD ENERGY Calories	PROTEIN Grams	FAT Grams	CARBO- HYDRATE Grams
Potatoes:				
Raw...	76	2.1	.1	17.1
Cooked:				
Baked in skin	93	2.6	.1	21.1
Boiled in skin	76	2.1	.1	17.1
Boiled, pared before cook-ing	65	1.9	.1	14.5
French-fried	274	4.3	13.2	36.0
Fried from raw	268	4.0	14.2	32.6
Hash-browned after hold-ing overnight	229	3.1	11.7	29.1
Mashed, milk added............	65	2.1	.7	13.0
Mashed, milk and table fat added	94	2.1	4.3	12.3
Scalloped and au gratin:				
With cheese	145	5.3	7.9	13.6
Without cheese...............	104	3.0	3.9	14.7
Canned:				
Solids and liquid...................	44	1.1	.2	9.8
Dehydrated mashed:				
Flakes without milk:				
Dry form...........................	364	7.2	.6	84.0
Prepared, water, milk, ta-ble fat added	93	1.9	3.2	14.5
Granules without milk:				
Dry form...........................	352	8.3	.6	80.4
Prepared, water, milk, ta-ble fat added	96	2.0	3.6	14.4
Granules with milk:				
Dry form..........................	358	10.9	1.1	77.7
Prepared, water, table fat added	79	2.0	2.2	13.1
Frozen:				
Diced, for hash-browning:				
Not thawed......................	73	1.2	Trace	17.4
Cooked, hash-browned....	224	2.0	11.5	29.0
French-fried:				
Not thawed......................	170	2.8	6.5	26.1
Heated...............................	220	3.6	8.4	33.7

FOOD AND DESCRIPTION *(per 100 grams, edible portion)*	FOOD ENERGY *Calories*	PROTEIN *Grams*	FAT *Grams*	CARBO-HYDRATE *Grams*
Mashed:				
Not thawed.......................	75	1.7	.1	17.1
Heated..............................	93	1.8	2.8	15.7
Potato chips	568	5.3	39.8	50.0
Potato flour	351	8.0	.8	79.9
Potato salad, from home recipe, made with—				
Cooked salad dressing, seasonings	99	2.7	2.8	16.3
Mayonnaise and French dressing, hard-cooked eggs, seasonings.	145	3.0	9.2	13.4
Potato sticks	544	6.4	36.4	50.8
Pretzels......................................	390	9.8	4.5	75.9
Pricklypears, raw...................	42	.5	.1	10.9
Prunes:				
Dehydrated, nugget-type and pieces:				
Uncooked	344	3.3	.5	91.3
Cooked, fruit and liquid, with added sugar	180	1.2	.2	47.1
Dried, "softenized":				
Uncooked	255	2.1	.6	67.4
Cooked (fruit and liquid):				
Without added sugar......	119	1.0	.3	31.4
With added sugar..........	172	.8	.2	45.1
Prune juice, canned or bottled	77	.4	.1	19.0
Prune whip	156	4.4	.2	36.9
Puddings with starch base, prepared from home recipe:				
Chocolate	148	3.1	4.7	25.7
Vanilla (blanc mange)	111	3.5	3.9	15.9
Pudding mixes and puddings made from mixes:				
With starch base:				
Mix, chocolate, regular, dry form	361	3.0	2.1	91.5
Pudding made with milk, cooked	124	3.4	3.0	22.8

FOOD AND DESCRIPTION (per 100 grams, edible portion)	FOOD ENERGY Calories	PROTEIN Grams	FAT Grams	CARBO-HYDRATE Grams
Mix, chocolate, instant, dry form	357	3.1	1.6	90.8
Pudding made with milk, without cooking	125	3.0	2.5	24.4
With vegetable gum base:				
Mix, custard-dessert, dry form	384	(0)	.1	98.9
Pudding made with milk, cooked	131	3.1	3.5	22.6
Pumpkin:				
Raw...	26	1.0	.1	6.5
Canned	33	1.0	.3	7.9
Pumpkin and squash seed kernels, dry	553	29.0	46.7	15.0
Radishes, raw:				
Common	17	1.0	.1	3.6
Oriental, including daikon (Japanese) and Chinese	19	.9	.1	4.2
Raisins, natural (unbleached):				
Uncooked	289	2.5	.2	77.4
Cooked, fruit and liquid, added sugar	213	1.2	.1	56.4
Raspberries:				
Raw:				
Black	73	1.5	1.4	15.7
Red	57	1.2	.5	13.6
Canned, solids and liquid, water pack, with or without artificial sweetener:				
Black	51	1.1	1.1	10.7
Red	35	.7	.1	8.8
Frozen, red, sweetened, not thawed	98	.7	.2	24.6
Rhubarb:				
Raw...	16	.6	.1	3.7
Cooked, added sugar..............	141	.5	.1	36.0
Frozen, sweetened:				
Not thawed..........................	75	.6	.2	18.5
Cooked, added sugar..........	143	.5	.2	36.2

FOOD AND DESCRIPTION (per 100 grams, edible portion)	FOOD ENERGY Calories	PROTEIN Grams	FAT Grams	CARBO-HYDRATE Grams
Rice:				
Brown:				
Raw......................................	360	7.5	1.9	77.4
Cooked	119	2.5	.6	25.5
White (fully milled or polished):				
Enriched:				
Common commercial varieties, all types:				
Raw	363	6.7	.4	80.4
Cooked..........................	109	2.0	.1	24.2
Long-grain:				
Parboiled:				
Dry form	369	7.4	.3	81.3
Cooked	106	2.1	.1	23.3
Precooked (instant):				
Dry form	374	7.5	.2	82.5
Ready-to-serve..........	109	2.2	Trace	24.2
Unenriched:				
Common commercial varieties, all types:				
Raw	363	6.7	.4	80.4
Cooked..........................	109	2.0	.1	24.2
Glutinous (Mochi Gomi), raw	361	5.6	.9	79.8
Rice bran	276	13.3	15.8	50.8
Rice polish.............................	265	12.1	12.8	57.7
Rice products used mainly as hot breakfast cereals:				
Rice, granulated, added nutrients:				
Dry form.............................	383	6.0	.3	85.9
Cooked	50	.8	Trace	11.2
Rice products used mainly as ready-to-eat breakfast cereals:				
Rice flakes, added nutrients..	390	5.9	.3	87.7
Rice, puffed; added nutrients, without salt	399	6.0	.4	89.5

FOOD AND DESCRIPTION (per 100 grams, edible portion)	FOOD ENERGY Calories	PROTEIN Grams	FAT Grams	CARBO-HYDRATE Grams
Rice, puffed or oven-popped, presweetened:				
Honey and added nutrients	388	4.2	.7	90.6
Honey or cocoa and added nutrients, including fat.	401	4.5	4.0	86.7
Rice, shredded; added nutrients	392	5.2	.3	88.8
Rice, with protein concentrate, mainly—				
Casein, other added nutrients	382	40.0	.2	54.8
Wheat gluten, other added nutrients	386	20.0	.3	74.4
Rice pudding with raisins	146	3.6	3.1	26.7
Rockfish, including black, canary, yellowtail, rasphead, and bocaccio:				
Raw..	97	18.9	1.8	0
Cooked, oven-steamed............	107	18.1	2.5	1.9
Roe:				
Raw:				
Including carp, cod, haddock, herring, pike, and shad.	130	24.4	2.3	1.5
Including salmon, sturgeon, and turbot	207	25.2	10.4	1.4
Cooked, baked or broiled, cod and shad	126	22.0	2.8	1.9
Canned, including cod, haddock, and herring, solids and liquid.	118	21.5	2.8	.3
Rolls and buns:				
Baked from home recipe, with milk and enriched flour.	339	8.2	8.7	56.1
Commercial:				
Ready-to-serve:				
Danish pastry..................	422	7.4	23.5	45.6
Hard rolls:				
Enriched	312	9.8	3.2	59.5
Unenriched	312	9.8	3.2	59.5
Plain (pan rolls):				

FOOD AND DESCRIPTION *(per 100 grams, edible portion)*	FOOD ENERGY Calories	PROTEIN Grams	FAT Grams	CARBO-HYDRATE Grams
Enriched	298	8.2	5.6	53.0
Unenriched	298	8.2	5.6	53.0
Raisin rolls or buns	275	6.9	2.9	56.4
Sweet rolls	316	8.5	9.1	49.3
Whole-wheat rolls	257	10.0	2.8	52.3
Partially baked (brown-and-serve):				
Enriched:				
Unbrowned	299	7.9	6.8	50.6
Browned	328	8.7	7.8	54.8
Unenriched:				
Unbrowned	299	7.9	6.8	50.6
Browned	328	8.7	7.8	54.8
Salad dressings, commercial:				
Blue and Roquefort cheese:				
Regular...............................	504	4.8	52.3	7.4
Special dietary (low-calorie):				
Low-fat (approx. 5 cal. per tsp.)	76	3.0	5.9	4.1
Low-fat (approx. 1 cal. per tsp.)	19	1.4	1.1	1.4
French:				
Regular................................	410	.6	38.9	17.5
Special dietary (low-calorie):				
Low-fat (approx. 5 cal. per tsp.)	96	.4	4.3	15.6
Low-fat with artificial sweetener (approx. 1 cal. per tsp.).	10	.4	.2	1.8
Medium-fat with artificial sweetener (approx. 10 cal. per tsp.).	156	.7	16.9	1.2
Italian:				
Regular...............................	552	.2	60.0	6.9
Special dietary (low-calorie, approx. 2 cal. per tsp.).	50	.2	4.7	2.6
Mayonnaise	718	1.1	79.9	2.2
Russian...................................	494	1.6	50.8	10.4

FOOD AND DESCRIPTION (per 100 grams, edible portion)	FOOD ENERGY Calories	PROTEIN Grams	FAT Grams	CARBO-HYDRATE Grams
Salad dressing (mayonnaise type):				
Regular............................	435	1.0	42.3	14.4
Special dietary (low-calorie, approx. 8 cal. per tsp.)	136	1.1	12.7	4.8
Thousand island:				
Regular............................	502	.8	50.2	15.4
Special dietary (low-calorie, approx. 10 cal. per tsp.).	180	.9	13.7	15.6
Salad dressings, made from home recipe:				
French............................	632	.3	70.1	3.6
Cooked	164	4.4	9.9	15.2
Salmon:				
Atlantic:				
Raw............................	217	22.5	13.4	0
Canned, solids and liquid ..	203	21.7	12.2	0
Chinook (king):				
Raw............................	222	19.1	15.6	0
Canned, solids and liquid ..	210	19.6	14.0	0
Chum:				
Raw............................	—	—	—	—
Canned, solids and liquid ..	139	21.5	5.2	0
Coho (silver):				
Raw............................	—	—	—	—
Canned, solids and liquid ..	153	20.8	7.1	0
Pink (humpback):				
Raw............................	119	20.0	3.7	0
Canned, solids and liquid ..	141	20.5	5.9	0
Sockeye (red):				
Raw............................	—	—	—	—
Canned, solids and liquid ..	171	20.3	9.3	0
Salmon, cooked, broiled or baked	182	27.0	7.4	0
Salmon rice loaf......................	122	12.0	4.5	7.3
Salmon, smoked	176	21.6	9.3	0
Sardines, Atlantic, canned in oil:				
Solids and liquid	311	20.6	24.4	.6
Drained solids	203	24.0	11.1	—

FOOD AND DESCRIPTION *(per 100 grams, edible portion)*	FOOD ENERGY *Calories*	PROTEIN *Grams*	FAT *Grams*	CARBO-HYDRATE *Grams*
Sardines, Pacific:				
Raw..	160	19.2	8.6	0
Canned:				
In brine or mustard, solids and liquid	196	18.8	12.0	1.7
In oil, drained solids	—	—	—	—
In tomato sauce, solids and liquid	197	18.7	12.2	1.7
Sauerkraut, canned, solids and liquid	18	1.0	.2	4.0
Sauerkraut juice, canned	10	.7	Trace	2.3
Sauger, raw	84	17.9	.8	0
Sausage, cold cuts, and luncheon meats:				
Blood sausage or blood pudding	394	14.1	36.9	.3
Bockwurst	264	11.3	23.7	.6
Bologna:				
All samples...........................	304	12.1	27.5	1.1
All meat	277	13.3	22.8	3.7
With nonfat dry milk	—	13.4	—	—
With cereal...........................	262	14.2	20.6	3.9
Braunschweiger......................	319	14.8	27.4	2.3
Brown-and-serve sausage:				
Before browning	393	13.5	36.0	2.7
Browned	422	16.5	37.8	2.8
Capicola or Capacola..............	499	20.2	45.8	0
Cervelat:				
Dry	451	24.6	37.6	1.7
Soft	307	18.6	24.5	1.6
Country-style sausage	345	15.1	31.1	0
Deviled ham, canned..............	351	13.9	32.3	0
Frankfurters:				
Raw:				
All samples......................	309	12.5	27.6	1.8
All meat	296	13.1	25.5	2.5
With nonfat dry milk......	300	13.1	25.6	3.4
With cereal	248	14.4	20.6	.2
With nonfat dry milk and cereal	—	14.2	21.7	—

FOOD AND DESCRIPTION (per 100 grams, edible portion)	FOOD ENERGY Calories	PROTEIN Grams	FAT Grams	CARBO- HYDRATE Grams
Cooked	304	12.4	27.2	1.6
Canned	221	13.4	18.1	.2
Headcheese	268	15.5	22.0	1.0
Knockwurst	278	14.1	23.2	2.2
Liverwurst:				
Fresh..................................	307	16.2	25.6	1.8
Smoked	319	14.8	27.4	2.3
Luncheon meat:				
Boiled ham	234	19.0	17.0	0
Pork, cured ham or shoul-der, chopped, spiced or unspiced, canned.	294	15.0	24.9	1.3
Meat loaf	200	15.9	13.2	3.3
Meat, potted (includes potted beef, chicken, and tur-key).	248	17.5	19.2	0
Minced ham	228	13.7	16.9	4.4
Mortadella	315	20.4	25.0	.6
Polish-style sausage	304	15.7	25.8	1.2
Pork and beef (chopped to-gether)	336	15.6	29.9	0
Pork sausage, links or bulk:				
Raw......................................	498	9.4	50.8	Trace
Cooked	476	18.1	44.2	Trace
Pork sausage, canned:				
Solids and liquid..................	415	13.8	38.4	2.4
Drained solids	381	18.3	32.8	1.9
Salami:				
Dry	450	23.8	38.1	1.2
Cooked	311	17.5	25.6	1.4
Scrapple	215	8.8	13.6	14.6
Souse....................................	181	13.0	13.4	1.2
Thuringer	307	18.6	24.5	1.6
Vienna sausage, canned	240	14.0	19.8	.3
Scallops, bay and sea:				
Raw......................................	81	15.3	.2	3.3
Cooked, steamed	112	23.2	1.4	—
Frozen, breaded, fried, re-heated	194	18.0	8.4	10.5
Shrimp:				
Raw......................................	91	18.1	.8	1.5

FOOD AND DESCRIPTION *(per 100 grams, edible portion)*	FOOD ENERGY Calories	PROTEIN Grams	FAT Grams	CARBO-HYDRATE Grams
Cooked, french-fried	225	20.3	10.8	10.0
Canned:				
Wet pack, solids and liquid	80	16.2	.8	.8
Dry pack or drained solids of wet pack	116	24.2	1.1	.7
Frozen, breaded, raw; not more than 50% breading	139	12.3	.7	19.9
Shrimp or lobster paste, canned	180	20.8	9.4	1.5
Sirups:				
Cane	263	0	0	68.
Maple	252	—	—	65.
Sorghum..................................	257	—	—	68.
Table blends:				
Chiefly corn, light and dark	290	0	0	75.
Cane and maple	252	0	0	65.
Soups, commercial:				
Canned:				
Asparagus, cream of:				
Condensed.........................	54	2.0	1.4	8.4
Prepared with equal volume of water	27	1.0	.7	4.2
Prepared with equal volume of milk	60	2.8	2.4	6.8
Bean with pork:				
Condensed.........................	134	6.4	4.6	17.3
Prepared with equal volume of water	67	3.2	2.3	8.7
Beef broth, bouillon, and consomme:				
Condensed.........................	26	4.2	0	2.2
Prepared with equal volume of water	13	2.1	0	1.1
Beef noodle:				
Condensed.........................	57	3.2	2.2	5.8
Prepared with equal volume of water	28	1.6	1.1	2.9
Celery, cream of:				
Condensed.........................	72	1.4	4.2	7.4
Prepared with equal volume of water	36	.7	2.1	3.7

FOOD AND DESCRIPTION (per 100 grams, edible portion)	FOOD ENERGY Calories	PROTEIN Grams	FAT Grams	CARBO- HYDRATE Grams
Prepared with equal volume of milk	69	2.6	3.8	6.2
Chicken consomme:				
Condensed.........................	18	2.8	.1	1.5
Prepared with equal volume of water	9	1.4	Trace	.8
Chicken, cream of:				
Condensed.........................	79	2.4	4.8	6.7
Prepared with equal volume of water	39	1.2	2.4	3.3
Prepared with equal volume of milk	73	3.0	4.2	5.9
Chicken gumbo:				
Condensed.........................	46	2.6	1.3	6.1
Prepared with equal volume of water	23	1.3	.6	3.1
Chicken noodle:				
Condensed.........................	53	2.8	1.6	6.6
Prepared with equal volume of water	26	1.4	.8	3.3
Chicken with rice:				
Condensed.........................	39	2.6	1.0	4.7
Prepared with equal volume of water	20	1.3	.5	2.4
Chicken vegetable:				
Condensed.........................	62	3.4	2.0	7.7
Prepared with equal volume of water	31	1.7	1.0	3.9
Clam chowder, Manhattan type (with tomatoes, without milk):				
Condensed.........................	66	1.8	2.1	10.0
Prepared with equal volume of water	33	.9	1.0	5.0
Minestrone:				
Condensed.........................	87	4.0	2.8	11.6
Prepared with equal volume of water	43	2.0	1.4	5.8
Mushroom, cream of:				
Condensed.........................	111	1.9	8.0	8.4

FOOD AND DESCRIPTION (per 100 grams, edible portion)	FOOD ENERGY Calories	PROTEIN Grams	FAT Grams	CARBO-HYDRATE Grams
Prepared with equal volume of water	56	1.0	4.0	4.2
Prepared with equal volume of milk	88	2.8	5.8	6.6
Onion:				
Condensed..........................	54	4.4	2.1	4.3
Prepared with equal volume of water	27	2.2	1.0	2.2
Pea, green:				
Condensed..........................	106	4.6	1.8	18.4
Prepared with equal volume of water	53	2.3	.9	9.2
Prepared with equal volume of milk	85	4.2	2.6	11.7
Pea, split:				
Condensed..........................	118	7.0	2.6	17.0
Prepared with equal volume of water	59	3.5	1.3	8.4
Tomato:				
Condensed..........................	72	1.6	2.1	12.7
Prepared with equal volume of water	36	.8	1.0	6.4
Prepared with equal volume of milk	69	2.6	2.8	9.0
Turkey noodle:				
Condensed..........................	65	3.6	2.4	7.0
Prepared with equal volume of water	33	1.8	1.2	3.5
Vegetable beef:				
Condensed..........................	65	4.2	1.8	7.9
Prepared with equal volume of water	32	2.1	.9	3.9
Vegetable with beef broth:				
Condensed..........................	64	2.2	1.4	11.0
Prepared with equal volume of water	32	1.1	.7	5.5
Vegetarian vegetable:				
Condensed..........................	64	1.8	1.7	10.6
Prepared with equal volume of water	32	.9	.8	5.4

FOOD AND DESCRIPTION (per 100 grams, edible portion)	FOOD ENERGY Calories	PROTEIN Grams	FAT Grams	CARBO-HYDRATE Grams
Dehydrated:				
Beef noodle:				
Mix, dry form..................	387	13.6	7.4	65.3
Prepared with 2 oz. mix in 3 cups water	28	1.0	.5	4.8
Chicken noodle:				
Mix, dry form..................	383	14.5	10.0	58.1
Prepared with 2 oz. mix in 4 cups water	22	.8	.6	3.2
Chicken rice:				
Mix, dry form..................	353	9.0	6.8	62.8
Prepared with 1½ oz. mix in 3 cups water	20	.5	.4	3.5
Onion:				
Mix, dry form..................	349	13.9	10.6	53.9
Prepared with 1½ oz. mix in 4 cups water	15	.6	.5	2.3
Pea, green:				
Mix, dry form..................	362	22.4	4.1	61.6
Prepared with 2 oz. mix in 3 cups water	50	3.1	.6	8.4
Tomato vegetable with noodles:				
Mix, dry form..................	348	8.7	8.0	62.7
Prepared with 2½ oz. mix in 4 cups water	27	.6	.6	5.1
Frozen:				
Clam chowder, New England type (with milk, without tomatoes):				
Condensed........................	107	3.7	6.4	8.6
Prepared with equal volume of water	54	1.8	3.2	4.4
Prepared with equal volume of milk	86	3.7	5.0	6.7
Pea, green, with ham:				
Condensed........................	113	7.6	2.3	16.0
Prepared with equal volume of water	57	3.8	1.2	8.0

FOOD AND DESCRIPTION *(per 100 grams, edible portion)*	FOOD ENERGY *Calories*	PROTEIN *Grams*	FAT *Grams*	CARBO-HYDRATE *Grams*
Potato, cream of:				
Condensed........................	87	2.7	4.3	10.0
Prepared with equal volume of water	44	1.4	2.2	4.9
Prepared with equal volume of milk	76	3.2	3.9	7.5
Shrimp, cream of:				
Condensed........................	133	4.0	9.9	7.2
Prepared with equal volume of water	66	2.0	5.0	3.5
Prepared with equal volume of milk	99	3.8	6.7	6.2
Vegetable with beef:				
Condensed........................	70	5.4	2.3	7.0
Prepared with equal volume of water	35	2.7	1.2	3.4
Soursop, raw	65	1.0	.3	16.3
Soybeans:				
Immature seeds:				
Raw	134	10.9	5.1	13.2
Cooked, boiled, drained	118	9.8	5.1	10.1
Canned:				
Solids and liquid..............	75	6.5	3.2	6.3
Drained solids..................	103	9.0	5.0	7.4
Mature seeds, dry:				
Raw	403	34.1	17.7	33.5
Cooked	130	11.0	5.7	10.8
Soybean milk:				
Fluid	33	3.4	1.5	2.2
Powder	429	41.8	20.3	28.0
Soybean milk products, sweetened:				
Liquid concentrate..................	126	4.8	7.3	12.3
Powder	452	20.4	23.2	48.4
Soybean protein	322	74.9	.1	15.1
Soybean proteinate	312	80.6	.1	7.7
Soy sauce	68	5.6	1.3	9.5
Spaghetti:				
Enriched:				
Dry form..............................	369	12.5	1.2	75.2

FOOD AND DESCRIPTION (per 100 grams, edible portion)	FOOD ENERGY Calories	PROTEIN Grams	FAT Grams	CARBO-HYDRATE Grams
Cooked, firm stage, "al dente" (8–10 min.)	148	5.0	.5	30.1
Cooked, tender stage (14–20 min.)	111	3.4	.4	23.0
Unenriched:				
Dry form	369	12.5	1.2	75.2
Cooked, firm stage, "al dente" (8–10 min.)	148	5.0	.5	30.1
Cooked, tender stage (14–20 min.)	111	3.4	.4	23.0
Spaghetti in tomato sauce with cheese:				
Cooked, from home recipe	104	3.5	3.5	14.8
Canned	76	2.2	.6	15.4
Spaghetti with meat balls in tomato sauce:				
Cooked, from home recipe	134	7.5	4.7	15.6
Canned	103	4.9	4.1	11.4
Spanish mackerel, raw	177	19.5	10.4	0
Spanish rice, cooked from home recipe	87	1.8	1.7	16.6
Spinach:				
Raw	26	3.2	.3	4.3
Cooked, boiled, drained	23	3.0	.3	3.6
Canned:				
Regular pack:				
Solids and liquid	19	2.0	.4	3.0
Drained solids	24	2.7	.6	3.6
Drained liquid	6	.5	0	1.3
Special dietary pack (low-sodium):				
Solids and liquid	21	2.5	.4	3.3
Drained solids	26	3.2	.5	4.0
Drained liquid	8	.5	0	2.0
Frozen:				
Chopped:				
Not thawed	24	3.1	.3	3.8
Cooked, boiled, drained ..	23	3.0	.3	3.7
Leaf:				
Not thawed	25	3.0	.3	4.2
Cooked, boiled, drained ..	24	2.9	.3	3.9

The Composition of Foods

FOOD AND DESCRIPTION (per 100 grams, edible portion)	FOOD ENERGY Calories	PROTEIN Grams	FAT Grams	CARBO-HYDRATE Grams
Squash:				
Summer:				
All varieties:				
Raw	19	1.1	0.1	4.2
Cooked, boiled, drained ..	14	.9	.1	3.1
Crookneck and Straightneck, Yellow:				
Raw	20	1.2	.2	4.3
Cooked, boiled, drained ..	15	1.0	.2	3.1
Scallop varieties, white and pale green:				
Raw	21	.9	.1	5.1
Cooked, boiled, drained ..	16	.7	.1	3.8
Zucchini and Cocozelle (Italian marrow type), green:				
Raw	17	1.2	.1	3.6
Cooked, boiled, drained ..	12	1.0	.1	2.5
Winter:				
All varieties:				
Raw	50	1.4	.3	12.4
Cooked:				
Baked.............................	63	1.8	.4	15.4
Boiled, mashed	38	1.1	.3	9.2
Acorn:				
Raw	44	1.5	.1	11.2
Cooked:				
Baked.............................	55	1.9	.1	14.0
Boiled, mashed	34	1.2	.1	8.4
Butternut:				
Raw	54	1.4	.1	14.0
Cooked:				
Baked.............................	68	1.8	.1	17.5
Boiled, mashed	41	1.1	.1	10.4
Hubbard:				
Raw	39	1.4	.3	9.4
Cooked:				
Baked.............................	50	1.8	.4	11.7
Boiled, mashed	30	1.1	.3	6.9
Squash, frozen:				
Summer, Yellow Crookneck:				

FOOD AND DESCRIPTION (per 100 grams, edible portion)	FOOD ENERGY Calories	PROTEIN Grams	FAT Grams	CARBO-HYDRATE Grams
Not thawed............................	21	1.4	.1	4.7
Cooked, boiled, drained	21	1.4	.1	4.7
Winter:				
Not thawed............................	38	1.2	.3	9.2
Heated....................................	38	1.2	.3	9.2
Squid, raw	84	16.4	.9	1.5
Stomach, pork, scalded............	152	16.5	9.0	0
Strawberries:				
Raw..	37	.7	.5	8.4
Canned, solids and liquid:				
Water pack, with or without artificial sweetener	22	.4	.1	5.6
Frozen, sweetened, not thawed:				
Sliced....................................	109	.5	.2	27.8
Whole	92	.4	.2	23.5
Sturgeon:				
Raw..	94	18.1	1.9	0
Cooked, steamed	160	25.4	5.7	0
Smoked....................................	149	31.2	1.8	0
Succotash (corn and lima beans), frozen:				
Not thawed	97	4.3	.4	21.5
Cooked, boiled, drained..........	93	4.2	.4	20.5
Sugars:				
Beet or cane:				
Brown	373	0	0	96.4
Granulated	385	0	0	99.5
Powdered	385	0	0	99.5
Dextrose:				
Anhydrous	366	0	0	99.5
Crystallized..........................	335	0	0	91.
Maple	348	—	—	90.
Sugarapples (sweetsop), raw..	94	1.8	.3	23.7
Sunflower seed kernels, dry	560	24.0	47.3	19.9
Sunflower seed flour, partially defatted	339	45.2	3.4	37.7
Swamp cabbage:				
Raw..	29	3.0	.3	5.4
Cooked, boiled, drained..........	21	2.2	.2	3.9

FOOD AND DESCRIPTION (per 100 grams, edible portion)	FOOD ENERGY Calories	PROTEIN Grams	FAT Grams	CARBO-HYDRATE Grams
Sweetbreads (thymus):				
Beef (yearlings):				
Raw	207	14.6	16.0	0
Cooked, braised	320	25.9	23.2	0
Calf:				
Raw	94	17.8	2.0	0
Cooked, braised	168	32.6	3.2	0
Lamb:				
Raw	94	14.1	3.8	0
Cooked, braised	175	28.1	6.1	0
Sweetpotatoes:				
Raw:				
All commercial varieties	114	1.7	.4	26.3
Firm-fleshed (Jersey types)	102	1.8	.7	22.5
Soft-fleshed (mainly Puerto Rico variety)	117	1.7	.3	27.3
Cooked, all:				
Baked in skin	141	2.1	.5	32.5
Boiled in skin	114	1.7	.4	26.3
Candied.................................	168	1.3	3.3	34.2
Canned:				
Liquid pack, solids and liquid:				
Regular pack in sirup	114	1.0	.2	27.5
Special dietary pack, without added sugar and salt.	46	.7	.1	10.8
Vacuum or solid pack	108	2.0	.2	24.9
Dehydrated flakes:				
Dry form..............................	379	4.2	.6	90.0
Prepared with water	95	1.0	.1	22.6
Swordfish:				
Raw..	118	19.2	4.0	0
Cooked, broiled	174	28.0	6.0	0
Canned, solids and liquid	102	17.5	3.0	0
Tamarinds, raw........................	239	2.8	.6	62.5
Tangelo juice, raw	41	.5	(.1)	9.7
Tangerines, raw (Dancy variety)	46	.8	.2	11.6

FOOD AND DESCRIPTION *(per 100 grams, edible portion)*	FOOD ENERGY Calories	PROTEIN Grams	FAT Grams	CARBO- HYDRATE Grams
Tangerine juice:				
Raw (Dancy variety)	43	.5	.2	10.1
Canned:				
Unsweetened	43	.5	.2	10.2
Sweetened............................	50	.5	.2	12.0
Frozen concentrate, unsweet- ened:				
Undiluted	162	1.7	(.7)	38.3
Diluted with 3 parts water, by volume	46	.5	(.2)	10.8
Tapioca, dry	352	.6	.2	86.4
Tapioca desserts:				
Apple tapioca	117	.2	.1	29.4
Tapioca cream pudding..........	134	5.0	5.1	17.1
Tomatoes, ripe:				
Raw..	22	1.1	.2	4.7
Cooked, boiled	26	1.3	.2	5.5
Canned, solids and liquid:				
Regular pack	21	1.0	.2	4.3
Special dietary pack (low- sodium)	20	1.0	.2	4.2
Tomato catsup, bottled	106	2.0	.4	25.4
Tomato chili sauce, bottled ..	104	2.5	.3	24.8
Tomato juice:				
Canned or bottled:				
Regular pack	19	.9	.1	4.3
Special dietary pack (low- sodium)	19	.8	.1	4.3
Canned concentrate:				
Undiluted	76	3.4	.4	17.1
Diluted with 3 parts water, by volume	20	.9	.1	4.5
Dehydrated (crystals):				
Dry form..............................	303	11.6	2.2	68.2
Prepared with water (1 lb. yields approx. 1¾ gals.).	20	.8	.1	4.5
Tomato juice cocktail, canned or bottled	21	.7	.1	5.0
Tomato paste, canned	82	3.4	.4	18.6
Tomato puree, canned:				

FOOD AND DESCRIPTION *(per 100 grams, edible portion)*	FOOD ENERGY Calories	PROTEIN Grams	FAT Grams	CARBO-HYDRATE Grams
Regular pack	39	1.7	.2	8.9
Special dietary pack (low-sodium)	39	1.7	.2	8.9
Tomcod, Atlantic, raw	77	17.2	.4	0
Tongue:				
Beef:				
Very fat, raw	271	14.4	23.	.4
Fat, raw	231	15.7	18.	.4
Medium-fat:				
Raw	207	16.4	15.	.4
Cooked, braised	244	21.5	16.7	.4
Thin (very thin), raw	175	17.4	11. .	.4
Smoked	—	17.2	28.8	—
Trout, brook, raw....................	101	19.2	2.1	0
Trout, rainbow or steelhead:				
Raw..	195	21.5	11.4	0
Canned	209	20.6	13.4	0
Tuna:				
Raw:				
Bluefin...................................	145	25.2	4.1	0
Yellowfin...............................	133	24.7	3.0	0
Canned:				
In oil:				
Solids and liquid..............	288	24.2	20.5	0
Drained solids..................	197	28.8	8.2	0
In water:				
Solids and liquid..............	127	28.0	.8	0
Tuna salad................................	170	14.6	10.5	3.5
Turkey:				
All classes:				
Total edible:				
Raw	218	20.1	14.7	0
Cooked, roasted	263	27.0	16.4	0
Flesh and skin:				
Cooked, roasted	223	31.9	9.6	0
Flesh only:				
Raw	162	24.0	6.6	0
Cooked, roasted	190	31.5	6.1	0
Skin only:				
Raw	405	12.1	39.2	0

FOOD AND DESCRIPTION *(per 100 grams, edible portion)*	FOOD ENERGY *Calories*	PROTEIN *Grams*	FAT *Grams*	CARBO-HYDRATE *Grams*
Cooked, roasted	451	17.0	42.0	0
Light meat:				
Raw	116	24.6	1.2	0
Cooked, roasted	176	32.9	3.9	0
Dark meat:				
Raw	128	20.9	4.3	0
Cooked, roasted	203	30.0	8.3	0
Giblets:				
Raw	150	20.1	6.6	1.2
Cooked (some gizzard fat), simmered	233	20.6	15.4	1.6
Veal:				
Carcass, raw:				
Including kidney and kidney fat:				
Fat class (76% lean, 24% fat)	248	18.0	19.	0
Medium-fat class (81% lean, 19% fat)	207	18.8	14.	0
Thin class (86% lean, 14% fat)	173	19.4	10.	0
Excluding kidney and kidney fat:				
Fat class (79% lean, 21% fat)	223	18.5	16.	0
Medium-fat class (84% lean, 16% fat)	190	19.1	12.	0
Thin class (88% lean, 12% fat)	156	19.7	8.	0
Retail cuts, untrimmed:				
Chuck:				
Fat class:				
Total edible, raw (83% lean, 17% fat)	198	19.0	13.	0
Medium-fat class:				
Total edible:				
Raw (86% lean, 14% fat)	173	19.4	10.	0
Cooked, braised (85% lean, 15% fat)	235	27.9	12.8	0

FOOD AND DESCRIPTION (per 100 grams, edible portion)	FOOD ENERGY Calories	PROTEIN Grams	FAT Grams	CARBO-HYDRATE Grams
Thin class:				
Total edible, raw (90% lean, 10% fat)	139	19.9	6.	0
Loin:				
Fat class:				
Total edible, raw (80% lean, 20% fat)	215	18.6	15.	0
Medium-fat class:				
Total edible:				
Raw (85% lean, 15% fat)	181	19.2	11.	0
Cooked, broiled (77% lean, 23% fat)	234	26.4	13.4	0
Thin class:				
Total edible, raw (89% lean, 11% fat)	156	19.7	8.	0
Rib:				
Fat class:				
Total edible, raw (76% lean, 24% fat)	248	18.0	19.	0
Medium-fat class:				
Total edible:				
Raw (82% lean, 18% fat)	207	18.8	14.	0
Cooked, roasted (82% lean, 18% fat)	269	27.2	16.9	0
Thin class:				
Total edible, raw (87% lean, 13% fat)	164	19.5	9.	0
Round with rump:				
Fat class:				
Total edible, raw (84% lean, 16% fat)	190	19.1	12.	0
Medium-fat class:				
Total edible:				
Raw (87% lean, 13% fat)	164	19.5	9.	0
Cooked, broiled (79% lean, 21% fat)	216	27.1	11.1	0

FOOD AND DESCRIPTION (per 100 grams, edible portion)	FOOD ENERGY Calories	PROTEIN Grams	FAT Grams	CARBO-HYDRATE Grams
Thin class:				
Total edible, raw (91% lean, 9% fat)	139	19.9	6.	0
Vegetable juice cocktail, canned	17	.9	.1	3.6
Vegetable main dishes, canned:				
Principal ingredients:				
Peanuts and soya................	237	11.7	16.9	13.4
Wheat protein	109	16.3	.8	8.8
Wheat protein, nuts or peanuts	212	20.3	7.1	17.7
Wheat protein, vegetable oil	189	19.1	10.4	5.2
Wheat and soy protein	104	16.1	1.2	7.6
Wheat and soy protein, soy or other vegetable oil	150	16.1	5.6	9.5
Vegetables, mixed (carrots, corn, peas, green snap beans, lima beans), frozen:				
Not thawed	65	3.3	.3	13.7
Cooked, boiled, drained..........	64	3.2	.3	13.4
Venison, lean meat only, raw	126	21.	4.	0
Vinegar:				
Cider	14	Trace	(0)	5.9
Distilled	12	—	—	5.
Vinespinach (basella), raw	19	1.8	.3	3.4
Waffles:				
Baked from home recipe, made with—				
Enriched flour	279	9.3	9.8	37.5
Unenriched flour	279	9.3	9.8	37.5
Frozen, made with enriched flour	253	7.1	6.2	42.0
Waffle mixes and waffles baked from mixes:				
Mix, with enriched flour, dry form	458	6.4	19.2	65.4
Waffles, made with water..	305	4.8	14.0	40.2

FOOD AND DESCRIPTION *(per 100 grams, edible portion)*	FOOD ENERGY Calories	PROTEIN Grams	FAT Grams	CARBO-HYDRATE Grams
Mix, with unenriched flour, dry form	458	6.4	19.2	65.4
Waffles, made with water ..	305	4.8	14.0	40.2
Mix (pancake and waffle), with enriched flour, dry form.	356	8.6	1.8	75.7
Waffles, made with egg, milk	275	8.8	10.6	36.2
Mix (pancake and waffle), with unenriched flour, dry form.	356	8.6	1.8	75.7
Waffles, made with egg, milk	275	8.8	10.6	36.2
Walnuts:				
Black.............................	628	20.5	59.3	14.8
Persian or English..................	651	14.8	64.0	15.8
Waterchestnut, Chinese (matai, waternut), raw	79	1.4	.2	19.0
Watercress leaves including stems, raw	19	2.2	.3	3.0
Watermelon, raw	26	.5	.2	6.4
Wheat bran, crude, commercially milled	213	16.0	4.6	61.9
Wheat germ, crude, commercially milled	363	26.6	10.9	46.7
Wheat products used mainly as hot breakfast cereals:				
Wheat, rolled:				
Dry form..............................	340	9.9	2.0	76.2
Cooked	75	2.2	.4	16.9
Wheat, whole-meal:				
Dry form..............................	338	13.5	2.0	72.3
Cooked	45	1.8	.3	9.4
Wheat and malted barley cereal, toasted:				
Quick-cooking:				
Dry form..........................	383	12.0	1.6	78.5
Cooked..............................	65	2.0	.3	13.2
Instant-cooking:				

FOOD AND DESCRIPTION (per 100 grams, edible portion)	FOOD ENERGY Calories	PROTEIN Grams	FAT Grams	CARBO-HYDRATE Grams
Dry form............................	382	14.0	1.6	76.2
Cooked..............................	80	3.0	.3	16.1
Wheat products used mainly as ready-to-eat breakfast cereals:				
Wheat flakes, added nutrients	354	10.2	1.6	80.5
Wheat germ, toasted..............	391	30.0	11.5	49.5
Wheat, puffed:				
Added nutrients, without salt	363	15.0	1.5	78.5
Added nutrients, with sugar and honey	376	6.0	2.1	88.3
Wheat, shredded:				
Without salt or other added ingredients	354	9.9	2.0	79.9
With malt, salt, and sugar added	366	9.1	2.9	81.7
Wheat and malted barley flakes, nutrients added	392	8.8	1.3	84.3
Wheat and malted barley granules, nutrients added	391	10.0	.6	84.4
Whey:				
Fluid	26	.9	.3	5.1
Dried.....................................	349	12.9	1.1	73.5
White sauce:				
Thin......................................	121	3.9	8.7	7.2
Medium.................................	162	3.9	12.5	8.8
Thick	198	4.0	15.6	11.0
Wildrice, raw	353	14.1	.7	75.3
Wreckfish, raw	114	18.4	3.9	0
Yam, tuber, raw........................	101	2.1	.2	23.2
Yambean, tuber, raw	55	1.4	.2	12.8
Yeast:				
Baker's:				
Compressed	86	(12.1)	.4	11.0
Dry (active)..........................	282	(36.9)	1.6	38.9
Brewer's, debittered	283	(38.8)	1.0	38.4
Torula	277	(38.6)	1.0	37.0

FOOD AND DESCRIPTION *(per 100 grams, edible portion)*	FOOD ENERGY *Calories*	PROTEIN *Grams*	FAT *Grams*	CARBO-HYDRATE *Grams*
Yellowtail (Pacific coast), raw	138	21.0	5.4	0
Yoghurt:				
Made from partially skimmed milk	50	3.4	1.7	5.2
Made from whole milk	62	3.0	3.4	4.9

INDEX